T0329892

COMPARING HEALTH SYSTEMS

Ian Greener

First published in Great Britain in 2021 by

Policy Press, an imprint of
Bristol University Press
University of Bristol
1–9 Old Park Hill
Bristol
BS2 8BB
UK
t: +44 (0)117 954 5940
e: bup-info@bristol.ac.uk

Details of international sales and distribution partners are available at
policy.bristoluniversitypress.co.uk

British Library Cataloguing in Publication Data
A catalogue record for this book is available from the British Library

ISBN 978-1-4473-5692-9 hardcover
ISBN 978-1-4473-5695-0 ePub
ISBN 978-1-4473-5694-3 ePdf

Cover design: Robin Hawes
Front cover image: iStock/bortonia
Bristol University Press and Policy Press use environmentally
responsible print partners.
Printed in Great Britain by TJ Books, Padstow

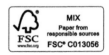

Contents

List of figures and tables   iv
Acknowledgements   vi

1   Introduction   1

2   Social determinants   29

3   Healthcare funding   62

4   Spending on health   93

5   COVID-19   115

6   Comparing health systems   128

7   Conclusion   141

Appendix: Method and data   154
Notes   165
References   166
Index   172

List of figures and tables

Figures

2.1	Life expectancy at birth, 2014	31
A1	Health expenditure calibration	158
A2	Behavioural factors calibration	158
A3	GINI coefficient calibration	159
A4	Pre-secondary education calibration	159
A5	Government health funding calibration	161
A6	Voluntary health insurance calibration	161
A7	Out-of-pocket funding calibration	162
A8	Curative and rehabilitative expenditure calibration	162
A9	Long-term care expenditure calibration	163
A10	Preventative care expenditure calibration	163

Tables

1.1	Social determinants of health for the 11 countries in the dataset	6
1.2	Health funding data for the 11 countries in the dataset	9
1.3	Health expenditure data for the dataset of 10 countries	12
1.4	Commonwealth Fund health outcomes scores	14
1.5	Commonwealth Fund health equity measures	15
1.6	Commonwealth Fund access measures	16
1.7	Commonwealth Fund efficiency scores	17
1.8	Commonwealth Fund care process scores	18
2.1	Social determinants calibrated dataset	34
2.2	Country clustering for the social determinants of health	35
2.3	Calibrated dataset for health outcomes	38
2.4	Truth table for social determinants and high health outcomes	39
2.5	Calibrated dataset for social determinants and high health equity	43
2.6	Truth table for social determinants and high health equity	44
2.7	Calibrated data for social determinants and high equity AND health outcomes	46
2.8	Truth table for social determinants and high health equity AND health outcomes	47
3.1	Calibrated fuzzy-set data for health funding in 11 countries	70
3.2	Fuzzy-set health funding clustering for 11 countries	71
3.3	High access and health funding fuzzy-set scores	72

3.4	Truth table for high health access and health funding	73
3.5	Calibrated dataset for high efficiency and health funding	75
3.6	Truth table for high health efficiency and health funding	77
3.7	Calibrated data for high access and efficiency, and health funding	79
3.8	Truth table for high access and efficiency, and health funding	80
4.1	Health expenditure calibrated dataset for 10 countries	99
4.2	Health expenditure truth table combinations	100
4.3	Calibrated health expenditure and high care scores	101
4.4	Truth table for high care scores and health expenditure	102
4.5	Calibrated dataset for high health outcomes and health expenditure	103
4.6	Truth table for high health outcomes and health expenditure	104
4.7	Calibrated dataset for high care and health outcomes and health expenditure for 10 countries	105
4.8	Truth table for high care and health outcomes, and health expenditure	106
5.1	COVID-19 contextual factors and testing for 25 OECD countries	119
5.2	Truth table for low COVID-19 mortality	120
6.1	Calibrated dataset for high health outcomes and key causal factors for 10 countries	130
6.2	Truth table for high health outcomes and key causal factors for 10 countries	131
6.3	Ranks of the 10 CF countries by health outcomes and PYLL	133
6.4	Calibrated dataset for PYLL and key causal factors for 31 countries (with US included twice)	135

Acknowledgements

Thanks to Linda, who put up with me writing this during lockdown in a pandemic. Thanks also to Adrian Dusa, for his endless patience in answering my questions about his R package that made the analysis possible, and to Emily, Beth and Joanna, for being themselves. In memory of Rupert, the greatest of all dogs, who was there at the beginning, but not the end, of this book. His legend will live on.

1

Introduction

This book compares the health systems of 11 countries in terms of their social determinants, health funding and health expenditure, and explores how the different configurations of these factors, in turn, relate to a range of different outcome measures. It also compares a wider range of countries in relation to the factors found most important for the 11 countries, as well as exploring the first-wave response to COVID-19 in 2020. By exploring health systems in terms of several of their most important aspects, we can assess what they have in common and in difference, and whether those commonalities and differences are linked to better or worse outcomes.

No empirical work takes place in a theoretical vacuum. Things that seem important are more likely to be measured, and those measures often already come in clusters, based on the relationships that we assume exist between them. It is therefore important to actively think about what it is we are trying to measure, what theories are explicit (or implicit) in those measures, and then whether the empirical findings that we find support or challenge those theories.

It is also really important in comparative research to have a method for linking together the existing data and theory, and for testing it in a robust and transparent manner. Not everyone will agree with the findings in this book, but they will be able to see exactly where they agree or disagree. I hope this can lead to debate, and in turn to greater understanding.

The starting point for the book is to identify what perspectives it will take – the different ways health systems will be explored – and, in outline, the debates that it will cover as a result. After that, this chapter moves on to consider the different outcomes each chapter will address, before explaining the method the book uses to achieve its comparative analysis.

Health systems

The dominant book on comparative health policy is that of Blank, Burau and Kuhlmann (2018), now in its fifth edition, which gives us an initial template for the topics or dimensions that this book should reasonably be expected to cover. Blank et al explore health policy in terms of its context, funding provision and governance, priorities and allocating resources, the health workforce, healthcare beyond the hospital, public health, and, finally, a chapter on exploring health policy comparatively. Across these chapters, the book presents a robust means of exploring different health systems, before its conclusion, which stresses the importance of breadth of coverage and the ability of the different frameworks and understandings in the book to 'map' (p 283) the different health systems of individual countries within it. Mapping means 'embracing complexity' to take a 'complex and dynamic view of health policy' that lacks 'the comfort that comes with the typology of health systems ... that it better reflects the real world of health care and its diverse actors' (p 283). I wholeheartedly share Blank et al's goals.

This book attempts to meet the challenge laid down by Blank et al, but also to extend its analysis in the following ways. It explores health systems from a range of different perspectives, most of which cut across the chapters presented in that book, while adopting an approach which acknowledges and embraces causal complexity. In order to achieve this, health systems are not treated in collections of simple causes and effects, but instead as configurations of causal factors which create rich contexts in different countries, with patterns of similarity and difference within them.

By combining different perspectives on health systems with causal complexity, the book aims to retain as much of the richness present in the health systems of different countries as possible, while at the same time looking for causal patterns within the configurations of factors present within them. It seeks to balance complexity with, where possible, generalisation by moving back and forward between causal factors and more detailed explorations of the health systems of different countries to try and learn as much as possible from the book's empirical analysis.

Any exploration of health systems needs to make a conscious choice about which countries to include in the analysis. If too many countries are included then there is a danger of over-abstraction so that the distinctive characteristics of the countries is lost. All the health systems risk merging into one another, and the specific characteristics and contexts within which health policy works can get lost. Including large numbers of countries also raises the risk of including countries in our comparisons which are not sufficiently alike. Although health policy is a global issue, it is hard to compare the health systems of very rich and poorer countries as they face different health challenges and have different levels of funding, staffing and infrastructure to call upon.

There is certainly scope for cross-national learning (World Health Organization, 2000), but systematic comparison between countries with high incomes, and those with much smaller economies and facing very different health challenges, is extremely difficult.

There is some excellent work comparing the health systems of a small number of countries, and this work brings rewards in terms of the depth of analysis and detail that can be accomplished. Immergut's (1992a) classic book compares health policymaking in France, Switzerland and Sweden, with a special focus on 'veto-points' in political processes, Moran's work on the 'Health Care State' (Moran, 1995, 1999) compares the UK, US and Germany in terms of their 'production', 'consumption' and 'regulation' systems, Tuohy's work (Tuohy, 1999) gives us rich insights into the development of the health systems in the US, Canada and the UK, and later expanded both her framework and range of countries to include the Netherlands (Tuohy, 2018); and Giamo's (2018) comparison of the US, Germany and South Africa gives real insight into the different challenges faced by those countries, giving us a new perspective on the challenge offered by HIV/AIDS in South Africa especially.

This book attempts to find a middle path between very large-scale, macro-comparative work, which can provide rigorous statistical analysis between countries, and the richness that smaller-scale comparisons between very small numbers of countries can provide. It explores the health systems of 11 countries. The countries are those included in the Commonwealth Fund's comparative measures of health systems (Schneider et al, 2017), not only because that gives us a unified basis for comparing their outcomes, but also because that sample covers a range of countries which are both diverse, but which also have a great deal in common. In the 11 countries (Australia, Canada, France, Germany, the Netherlands, Norway, New Zealand, Sweden, Switzerland, the UK and the US) there are countries which are at broadly the same level of economic development (but which spend very different amounts on their health systems), which have established health systems (but with significant differences in their organisation), and which cover a significant part of the world – including North America, Europe and Australasia.

The coverage of the countries fits well with existing typologies of welfare and health systems, as well as having geographical justification. In relation to Esping-Andersen's '3 worlds' typology of welfare states (Esping-Andersen, 1990) Australia, Canada, New Zealand, the UK and the US represent the 'liberal' type, France, Germany and Switzerland are 'conservative', and the Netherlands, Norway and Sweden are 'social democratic'. This means the 11 countries allow comparisons between all three welfare worlds. In relation to a more recent typology of health systems, that of Reibling et al (2019) Switzerland and the US are 'supply and performance – private', Australia, France and Germany are 'supply and choice – public', Norway, New Zealand and Sweden are 'performance and primary care – public', and Canada, the Netherlands and the UK are 'regulation public systems'. The countries therefore represent four of the five clusters in Reibling's typology, with the 'low supply and low performance – mixed' not covered, but with the countries listed under that type (Estonia, Hungary, Poland and Slovakia) often being at the limits of the measures of the different factors that are included in the book, and stretching the limits of comparison as a result.

There are of course gaps in relation to this country coverage – but the sample includes a great deal of diversity which can be put to good use in exploring differences (and similarities) across the countries, while at the same time having sufficient detail about each of the countries to retain their own distinctive individual character. As such, the Commonwealth Fund's 11 countries have sufficient in common to make them comparable, while at the same time having a good range of diversity of different health and welfare system types. This means that the book's comparisons should be between countries facing similar health challenges, but which have made different choices about their approach to healthcare and health policy.

As well justifying the choice of countries in the book, there is also a need to explain the elements or dimensions of health systems that will be included here. The book explores the social determinants of health, health funding, health expenditure, and, in a separate chapter, a range of factors relevant to the first-wave COVID-19 response. The next section explains those choice and outlines the data which will be used.

The social determinants of health

Chapter 2 considers health systems in terms of the social determinants of health. Putting social determinants first makes clear that what goes on in health systems is not only located in their healthcare systems, but that it is also crucial to understand the effects of a range of other factors, including levels of inequality, education levels, and behavioural factors such as smoking and drinking. By looking for patterns of these factors across our countries, the book can begin to explore the different challenges the 11 countries face, and so construct a first comparison in terms of their social determinants.

The different social determinants of health included in the book are outlined fully in Chapter 2. However, in brief, the factors included are health expenditure, income inequality, a measure of the population with pre-secondary education, and a combined index of drinking and smoking.

Health expenditure is such an important causal factor that it is present in all the chapters of the book because of existing research showing its importance to all the outcome measures included (Deaton, 2015; OECD, 2017). In terms of the social determinants, there are a wide range of possible additional factors, but there is a consensus that we should consider levels of inequality as being important, especially in the work of Michael Marmot (Marmot and Wilkinson, 2005; Marmot, 2012, 2015), who identifies a 'health gap' between countries with lower and higher levels of inequality. Inequality, however, is not the only factor we should consider – education levels are important, as they are often linked to opportunity, and because people who are more highly educated should, at least in theory, be able to make better decisions about their own health. Equally, we now know that people who have pre-secondary (in UK terms) education levels only are much more susceptible to 'deaths of despair' (Case and Deaton, 2020) stemming from the lack of esteem in which their lives and work appear to be held in increasingly meritocratic societies (Sandel, 2020). At the same time, there are behavioural factors which are now well understood as potentially reducing health outcomes, with smoking and higher levels of drinking often identified as having particularly damaging effects (OECD, 2017).

The measures for the social determinants outlined earlier are shown in Table 1.1.

In Table 1.1, GINI is the GINI income inequality measure (post taxes and transfers), TOB is the proportion of people who are smokers, ALC is average alcohol consumption per year (in litres), HEALTHEXP is expenditure on healthcare in US$ PPP, and EDUC is the proportion of the population educated to pre-comprehensive level only.

There are some immediately striking things about Table 1.1. The US has the highest GINI measure (and so has the highest degree of income inequality), and by far the highest level of health expenditure, but its levels of tobacco and alcohol consumption, and its numbers of people with lower levels of education, are low. Norway and Sweden both have lower levels of income inequality than the other countries. The proportion of people smoking tobacco consumption is in the 20s in France, Germany and Switzerland, but with Sweden and the US being much lower. Levels of alcohol consumption also appear high in France and Germany compared to other countries. The education measure

Table 1.1: Social determinants of health for the 11 countries in the dataset

COUNTRY	GINI	TOB	ALC	HEALTHEXP	EDUC
Australia	0.33	13.00	9.70	4708.09	21.00
Canada	0.31	14.00	8.10	4752.78	9.60
France	0.29	22.40	11.90	4600.36	22.50
Germany	0.29	20.90	11.00	5550.63	13.20
Netherlands	0.29	19.00	8.00	5385.41	23.60
New Zealand	0.35	15.00	8.70	3589.59	25.30
Norway	0.26	13.00	6.00	6647.46	17.60
Sweden	0.28	11.20	7.20	5487.52	18.00
Switzerland	0.30	20.40	9.50	7919.02	12.70
UK	0.35	17.80	9.50	4192.46	20.40
US	0.39	11.40	8.80	9892.25	10.50

considers the proportion of people with low levels of education, so a lower number here should lead to better outcomes. Canada and the US appear to have the lowest results, whereas New Zealand, the Netherlands and France's results are much higher.

Even a quick inspection of Table 1.1, then, leads to some interesting questions – are the relatively low measures for tobacco, alcohol and education in the US, along with its high health expenditure, enough to overcome any health outcome problems that might result from its very high GINI coefficient? At the other end, is the low GINI measure for France enough to overcome any problems that might result from high tobacco and alcohol consumption, and from it having a large number of people with low levels of education? How do these dynamics play out in the other countries and with other combinations of social determinants?

By considering how these factors – health expenditure, inequality, education levels, and smoking and drinking – interrelate, it is possible to explore how countries compare across these factors, as well as beginning to see whether particular patterns of these factors seems to be linked to better or worse outcomes. If differences in health outcomes are often empirically linked to differences in health expenditure on average, how does this play out in the 11 countries explored here, taking the other factors into account as well? Are differences in health outcomes most related to patterns with behavioural factors such as levels of smoking or drinking, or higher-level factors such as inequality?

Chapter 2 considers the social determinants of health. Chapter 3 moves onto the issue of how healthcare should be funded.

Health funding

How health systems are funded is often taken for granted within individual countries, but if the issue is considered comparatively, then it quickly becomes clear that the policymakers of different countries have come up with very different approaches to paying for health services.

In broad terms, there are three options, but with considerable variation between health systems on the emphasis and balance between them. First, people needing access to health services can pay for them from their own funds, or in the language of the Organisation for Economic Co-operation and Development (OECD), we can fund them 'out-of-pocket'. Policymakers might like this option because it links funding with willingness to pay in a very explicit way. Even where people do not pay the full cost of their treatment, the use of out-of-pocket payments can prevent the overuse of services that can result if people are covered by health insurance policies, or health services are funded by the government. The use of out-of-pocket payments is often based on the idea that people should at least partially contribute to healthcare cost from their own funds, and is often combined with systems of means testing or requirements that people 'co-pay' the costs of healthcare in some form. Opponents of out-of-pocket payments, however, suggest they may end up leading to people deciding not to visit health services when they need to – especially where those people are relatively poor.

The second OECD headline form of health funding comes through the use of health insurance, in which individuals or employers might pay into a scheme to try and ensure that, should people (or perhaps their families) fall ill, the funds will be available to pay for their care. Health insurance can be voluntary, where people choose whether they want to take it out or not, or compulsory, whereby the government has decided that everyone should be covered in order to make sure everyone can access health services if they need to. The OECD and World Health Organization categorise the two separately, with compulsory health insurance being regarded as similar to government funding (from taxation) health systems (OECD et al, 2017). This marks an important distinction because all the health systems here have significant levels of government and compulsory insurance funding to attempt to address the problem of what should be done where people are unable to pay for healthcare that they need out of pocket, and also do not hold voluntary health insurance.

The third means of funding healthcare is where it is paid for by the government, or by compulsory health insurance. Systems based on government or compulsory health insurance attempt to ensure that everyone in a country can access at least some form of healthcare should they need to. Advocates of funding healthcare through government and compulsory health insurance argue that the very high cost of healthcare, and the significant role of luck in whether we require healthcare or not, mean that 'risk pooling' – creating a fund into which everyone pays at different rates, but from which they can also draw funding should they need to – is the fairest way to fund health systems.

All the countries included in the book have a balance between these three means of healthcare funding, with countries that prefer a more solidaristic approach, and which regard access to healthcare as a universal right, tending towards a system which has a larger government and compulsory insurance component. Countries which regard people as needing to take greater responsibility for their own healthcare will still have government and/or compulsory insurance, but tend to have a greater element of voluntary health insurance, reserving government funding only for those that cannot afford to pay for healthcare themselves. Out-of-pocket expenditures are used to some extent by all the countries here, but tend to be larger when countries make extensive use of means testing, perhaps to encourage more the responsible use of health services, or as a way of increasing the overall funding available for health services where it may be difficult to increase taxation or raise insurance premiums further.

Implicit in different forms of health funding are debates around ensuring people have appropriate access to health services, but which are also linked to issues around personal responsibility and what is the most efficient means of providing health funding – an issue that has come more and more to the fore as the costs of healthcare have increased.

The OECD statistics for health financing included in the book are presented in Table 1.2.

In Table 1.2, two HEALTHEXP refers to health expenditure per capita (US$), GOV to the percentage of total health funding from government or compulsory insurance, VOL the percentage of total health funding from voluntary health insurance, and OOP the mean per capita (US$) payment for out-of-pocket expenditures.

There are some striking initial patterns in the data. Again, the US appears as an outlier because of its very high health expenditure (as

Table 1.2: Health funding data for the 11 countries in the dataset

COUNTRY	HEALTHEXP	GOV	VOL	OOP
Australia	4708.09	67.75	12.61	838.81
Canada	4752.78	70.29	15.31	672.81
France	4600.36	78.83	7.25	307.87
Germany	5550.63	84.58	2.59	670.60
Netherlands	5385.41	80.84	7.27	648.94
New Zealand	3589.59	80.20	7.84	429.67
Norway	6647.46	85.21	0.48	883.49
Sweden	5487.52	83.89	1.17	800.04
Switzerland	7919.02	63.62	7.63	2136.02
UK	4192.46	79.19	6.18	610.31
US	9892.25	49.13	39.79	1053.77

noted under social determinants), but also because of its proportionally low level of government expenditure. The figures for the US treat the changes made by the Affordable Care Act (ACA or 'Obamacare') as not introducing compulsory health insurance. Whether the ACA represents compulsory or voluntary health insurance is a complex matter, with the OECD treating it as such from 2016 onwards, but the Commonwealth Fund not doing so, and with things still very much in flux at the time of the book's writing because of the uneven implementation of the ACA. However, beyond definitional disputes, because health systems, and especially health outcomes, take a great deal of time to change, it made more sense to reflect the situation in the US as the OECD measured it up to 2017, rather than trying to measure the different pattern of funding which is now in place, but will have had relatively little effect yet.

Looking beyond the US, Norway and Sweden have the highest levels of government and compulsory insurance expenditure, and also the lowest levels of voluntary health insurance. More generally, government and compulsory insurance makes up the largest share of health funding for all the systems here, including even the US. The US, Canada and Australia have the highest levels of voluntary health insurance, with the US being by far the highest of the three. In terms of out-of-pocket funding, Switzerland has by far the highest levels, followed by the US, but with Sweden and Norway also having relatively high levels, which does not entirely fit with the characterisation of their systems as being social democratic in nature (Kenworthy, 2019).

Health expenditure

Chapter 4 considers the area of health expenditure. The logic here is that, after considering the factors which fall outside the direct control of health services (social determinants), then at the different ways health services are funded, it then makes sense to consider what that money is spent on.

There are at least two approaches that the book could take to the question of expenditure. The first looks at the different high-level expenditure categories present in health services used in health accounting systems to try and get comparable data, and which measure, in broad terms, the balance of expenditures between acute (urgent), long-term and preventative healthcare categories. The second approach would be to look at how health expenditures result in expenditures on different categories of health professionals, along with other factors such as the numbers of hospitals beds to see if particular skills mixes seem to work better than others. The original plan for the book was to do both. And then COVID-19 appeared, and so there was clearly a need for a book on comparative health systems to address the responses of countries to the pandemic – thus that will be the topic of Chapter 5. Although the analysis for both expenditure and skills mixes was carried out, the expenditure chapter has more interesting and challenging findings, and so that chapter has been retained. As such, Chapter 4 considers health expenditures in terms of the high-level categories from the OECD.

Health expenditure carries with it some almost directly conflicting theories about the right way to spend money on healthcare, which are born of the tensions that politicians and policymakers face in running health services. On the one hand, there is a clear imperative to make sure that as much money as possible is spent on the current health needs of their public – and this tends to be on health services designed to look after illnesses and injuries that need to be addressed now. If people are waiting too long to be treated, or are unable to access health services at all, this has the potential to cause real harm to them, and also to generate adverse publicity for politicians and policymakers, especially where it involves particular groups, such as children, which are likely to capture media interest. Politicians have rational reasons for wanting to increase expenditure on health services which are focused on 'cure', either by providing more services designed to address this, or for increased funding for new drugs or treatments.

However, health expenditure can also be for a range of other purposes. As life expectancies increase, many more of us require long-term care, which may never fully cure us of conditions such as asthma or arthritis, but instead aim to make life as liveable as possible with such conditions, and perhaps to prevent further deterioration. So there is a tension between curative and long-term expenditure, with every country spending much more on the former, but with some prepared to reallocate greater expenditures to the latter.

In addition to long-term care, there is also preventative healthcare expenditure. This area, which can be contentious as it can be regarded by some people as the 'nanny state' telling them 'what to do', is responsible for considering collective healthcare issues, such as smoking, drinking and diet, but also issues such as vaccinations and screenings. Much of the emphasis will be on attempting behavioural change in the case of lifestyle, or compliance in the case of vaccination and screening programmes. Spending in this area is designed to prevent health problems in the future – but because of the (in some eyes) paternalistic messages being presented here, and because improvements may take years and years to appear and so are difficult to measure, preventative healthcare expenditures are sometimes regarded with suspicion. Increasing expenditure on preventative care, as with long-term care, means moving resources from curative healthcare, where services may already be hard pressed, but requires an even braver politician or policymaker as the results of expenditure here are unlikely to appear during their own political careers owing to the likely time lags involved.

The data for the book, which cover 10 countries only as New Zealand does not comply with the OECD's reporting measures for health expenditures, are presented in Table 1.3.

In Table 1.3, HEALTHEXP, is health expenditure, CUREREHAB is the percentage of health expenditure on curative and rehabilitative services, LONG is the percentage of health expenditure on long-term care, and PREVENT is the percentage of health expenditure on preventative healthcare.

Looking at the data, the very large difference in expenditures between the US and the other countries of the world is again apparent, but in the particular configuration here the US spends the second-highest on curative and rehabilitative expenditure, but the second-lowest on long-term care, and what appears to be a middling percentage of expenditure on preventative care. It is also clear that preventative care is by far the lowest area of spend for most countries here, except for Australia, which appears to spend massively less on long-term care than other countries while having the highest proportion of spend on curative and rehabilitative expenditure. The Netherlands, Norway and Sweden are the highest spenders on long-term care, while also being

Table 1.3: Health expenditure data for the dataset of 10 countries

COUNTRY	HEALTHEXP	CUREREHAB	LONG	PREVENT
Australia	4708.09	63.6	1.2	1.8
Canada	4752.78	46.2	16.2	5.8
France	4600.36	45.7	14.4	2.0
Germany	5550.63	49.1	14.9	3.2
Netherlands	5385.41	46.0	25.7	4.3
Norway	6647.46	48.3	28.5	2.6
Sweden	5487.52	49.9	26.3	3.5
Switzerland	7919.02	53.4	19.3	2.6
UK	4192.46	49.4	18.7	5.1
US	9892.25	61.9	5.7	3.3

among the highest in terms of overall spend. The UK and Canada have the highest preventative care spends, and both are towards the lower end of overall expenditure and seem comparable in terms of curative and long-term expenditure.

COVID-19

Exploring different countries' responses to COVID-19 was not in the original book proposal as that was presented to the publishers well before the pandemic began. However, most of the book was written during 2020 and it became increasingly clear that not discussing the pandemic in a book on comparative health systems would have been a significant omission. At the same time, because the pandemic was still far from over by the time the chapter had to be written (in September and October 2020), it could not present a final view on it.

The chapter on COVID-19 uses different data from the rest of the book, considering factors identified in the pandemic as being causally important in COVID-19 mortality (obesity rates, age, and a measure of deprivation) along with a measure used in Economist Intelligence Unit work as a proxy for the openness of a country at the beginning of the pandemic – international arrivals. It takes these data in mid-July 2020, when the first wave of the pandemic was over for most countries, as a means of assessing the initial situations and response to COVID-19 for 25 OECD countries (those for which full datasets could be compiled). In terms of response, the chapter uses a measure of COVID-19 tests per COVID-19 case, which was shown to be an important factor in generating solutions. In terms of outcomes, the chapter assesses the success of different countries in terms of both their COVID-19 mortality and COVID-19 case rates, and then in terms of the countries that have had comparative success in terms of both of these factors.

Comparing health systems

Finally, the book takes key factors identified in the chapters exploring social determinants, health funding and health expenditure, and puts them together to compare health systems based upon them, both in terms of the sample of countries in Chapters two, three and four, but also expanding the range of countries to 31 to test whether the factors (albeit with a slightly different outcome measure for the expanded range of countries) work with an expanded dataset as well.

Health outcomes

In the causal factor sections covering Chapters 2, 3 and 4 (social determinants, health funding and health expenditure) the related outcomes the book will be investigating were not directly mentioned. This section explains the choice of outcome measures for each of those chapters.

Social determinants outcomes

In terms of the social determinants of health, the book explores how the patterns of causal factors (inequality, health expenditure, alcohol, tobacco, education) are related to two outcome factors from the Commonwealth Fund report. The first of these is health outcomes. This is a measure combining a complex range of measures from population health (infant mortality, number of adults with at least two chronic conditions, life expectancy at age 60), mortality amenable to healthcare, and disease-specific health outcomes for a range of common conditions. Each country is graded across these measures, and their score standardised across the 11 countries and averaged.

The Commonwealth Fund's health outcomes scores (where higher numbers are better) for 2017 are shown in Table 1.4.

In Table 1.4, there is a range of final ratings, from 0.62 (the highest, Australia), to 0.55 (Sweden) and 0.42 (Norway), down to −0.63 (UK) and −0.76 (US). These standardised scores have a 'centre' of 0, so that countries performing better than their peers have a score above 0, and

Table 1.4: Commonwealth Fund health outcomes scores

COUNTRY	SCORE
Australia	0.62
Canada	−0.35
France	0.23
Germany	−0.18
Netherlands	0.03
New Zealand	−0.12
Norway	0.42
Sweden	0.55
Switzerland	0.32
UK	−0.63
US	−0.76

those worse have scores below zero. This means the Netherlands falls just in the set of countries performing well – with a score of 0.03.

Exploring the social determinants of health in relation to health outcomes allows the book to systematically explore whether there appears to be a relationship between the two. Do countries that are performing well according to the health outcomes measure have patterns of social determinants that advocates of reducing inequalities would expect, or are they more closely linked to behavioural factors or education levels? Are they much more related to levels of health expenditure instead?

In addition to the social determinants of health in relation to health outcomes, the book also considers them in terms of their relationship to the Commonwealth Fund's measure of health equity. This measure compares the indicators across a range of domains to assess the gap between those on above-average and below-average incomes. The bigger the differences found, the less equitable the health system is judged to be. With this in mind, the measure considers these differences in terms of surveys about patient satisfaction in relation to treatment, whether consultations about diet and exercise were taking place, as well as access to medical history, patient engagement, affordability, and the timeliness of treatment. This leads to the results shown in Table 1.5.

As such, these results show a scale from 0.93 (UK) down to −0.94 (US), with Germany just being in the set of countries with high health equity (0.01).

Table 1.5: Commonwealth Fund health equity measures

COUNTRY	SCORE
Australia	−0.14
Canada	−0.39
France	−0.53
Germany	0.01
Netherlands	0.46
New Zealand	−0.24
Norway	0.14
Sweden	0.37
Switzerland	0.34
UK	0.93
US	−0.94

Comparing the two tables of outcome measures, health outcomes (Table 1.4) and equity (Table 1.5), some countries score well on both measures (the Netherlands, Norway, Sweden, Switzerland), and others score poorly on both (Canada, New Zealand, US). Some countries, like the UK, score poorly on outcomes, but very well on equity. These contrasts give us the opportunity to consider countries in terms of both sets of outcomes, which in the set-theoretical logic used in the book, means countries are assessed in terms of their lower score of the two, or the weakest link in terms of the two outcomes. So, as well as exploring health outcomes and health equity, the book also explores patterns of social determinants compared to the minimum score for those two outcomes to see what this reveals about the health systems which are most able to achieve that demanding measure.

Health funding outcomes

In terms of health funding, the book uses two different Commonwealth Fund outcome measures, those for access and those for administrative efficiency.

The access measure is divided in two subdomains, which measure the affordability timeliness of health services. Affordability measures a range of issues in respect of cost-related access, including whether appointments were skipped due to costs, if insurance claims were denied, and the extent of patient and doctor reports of problems paying medical bills. Timeliness measures whether a regular doctor is

Table 1.6: Commonwealth Fund access measures

COUNTRY	SCORE
Australia	0.19
Canada	−0.77
France	−0.14
Germany	0.58
Netherlands	0.70
New Zealand	0.02
Norway	0.14
Sweden	0.06
Switzerland	−0.11
UK	0.39
US	−1.07

available, how difficult after-hours care is to access, as well as waiting times in emergency rooms, and waits for tests and treatments. The two scores are then standardised and averaged to produce the results shown in Table 1.6.

Here there is a range of scores going from 0.7 (Netherlands) and 0.58 (Germany) down to Canada (−0.77) and the US −1.07), with New Zealand just falling into the high access set of countries (0.02).

Health service administrative efficiency many not seem a very glamorous outcome goal, but in terms of health funding it is essential. Health services are around 10 per cent of all the spending in the economy in most of the countries here (for some, like the US, much more). Efficiency is crucial as, because health spending makes up such a large share of government spending, spending money poorly on health services results in less funding for other public services as well as for other health services.

The administrative efficiency Commonwealth Fund measure is made up of a range of different indicators assessing doctor time spent on payment claims, doctor time spent on getting patients medications, doctor time spent on other administration, patients visiting emergency rooms when they should have gone through other routes for their care, slow test results, a measure of unnecessary testing, and time spent on medical bill paperwork or disputes. After standardisation and averaging, the results in Table 1.7 are generated.

Here then is a range of values from 0.74 (Australia), 0.6 (New Zealand) and 0.59 (UK), through to −1.21 (US) and −1.41 (France).

Table 1.7: Commonwealth Fund efficiency scores

COUNTRY	SCORE
Australia	0.74
Canada	0.08
France	−1.41
Germany	0.08
Netherlands	−0.15
New Zealand	0.60
Norway	0.54
Sweden	0.26
Switzerland	−0.12
UK	0.59
US	−1.21

Finally, in terms of the outcomes related to health funding, the book looks at both access and efficiency by considering the lowest score each country has achieved on either measure. Australia, Germany, New Zealand, Norway, Sweden and the UK have positive scores for both access and efficiency, whereas France, Switzerland and the US have negative scores for both measures.

Health expenditure outcomes

For health expenditure the book explores patterns of overall expenditure levels (in common with the chapters on social determinants and health funding), along with curative, long-term and preventative expenditure, using the Commonwealth Fund care process and health outcomes measures. The logic for using the care process measure is that it is surely important that health expenditures lead to better care, and so finding out if this is the case is a crucial question.

The Commonwealth Fund care process measures are the most complex of all its indicators, spanning a range of nine different measures of preventative care, three measures of safe care, seven measures of coordinated care, and 10 measures of engagement and patient preferences. The standardised and averaged measures shown in Table 1.8.

Care process measures range from 0.56 (UK) down to −0.82 (Sweden), with Switzerland just falling into the set of countries with low care outcomes (−0.03). These scores are immediately surprising

Table 1.8: Commonwealth Fund care process scores

COUNTRY	SCORE
Australia	0.38
Canada	0.15
France	−0.42
Germany	−0.12
Netherlands	0.29
Norway	−0.60
Sweden	−0.82
Switzerland	−0.03
UK	0.56
US	0.23

considering the success of Sweden and Switzerland in other outcome measures in the book, and because the US has a positive score here for the first time.

As well as measuring the relationship between different forms of health expenditure and care process, the book also explores the relationship between expenditures and health outcomes, to explore whether the tensions we identified earlier – especially between patterns of curative, long-term and preventative expenditure – lead to differences in health outcomes.

As such, the book uses the Commonwealth Fund measure of health outcomes twice – first for social determinants, and then again for health expenditure. This may seem strange, but there are two justifications for that choice.

The first reason is that, in choosing health outcomes for both social determinants and health expenditures, different perspectives on health are being taken. The social world is complex, and one set of causal factors (either social determinants or health expenditure) cannot fully account for something as complex as health outcomes. In taking different perspectives, the ability to understand how both sets of causal factors contribute to health outcomes is enhanced.

The second reason is that exploring outcomes using different causal factors fits within the logic of the method used in the book. That logic is based around set-theoretical understandings, where sufficient solutions between sets of causal factors and one outcome do not mean that outcome is fully explained as there can still be other means of achieving the outcome, or through combinations of other causal factors. Exploring health outcomes as they relate to social determinants does not preclude their being explored in relation to health expenditure factors as well. The Appendix to the book explores its method in depth, but an outline also appears in the next section.

Qualitative Comparative Analysis

This book's main method for comparing health systems is fuzzy-set QCA (Qualitative Comparative Analysis). QCA is a configurational method designed by Charles Ragin (Ragin, 2000, 2008, 2014) and developed further by Ragin himself, along with methodologists such as Scheider and Waggeman (2012) and Dusa (2018). It aims to provide a rigorous means of comparing configurations of causal factors and how they relate to outcomes, finding patterns in datasets based on set-theoretical logic. It is a mixed-method strategy which involves going back and forward between the individual cases (here, the health systems) and the results (the configurations of causal factors and outcomes), to improve understanding of how the measures illuminate our knowledge of the cases, and how detailed knowledge of the cases can help us interpret the measures.

A description of QCA as a method, and the exact method by which it was applied may be found in the Appendix to the book, but an outline can be given here.

Fuzzy-set QCA is a method which is designed to find a middle way between quantitative and qualitative analysis in that it applies an, in principle, repeatable and rigorous method for cross-analysing cases, while at the same time allowing detailed case-based knowledge to be assembled and applied. Cases are explored in terms of how their configurations of causal factors (social determinants, health funding, health expenditure, and factors associated with COVID) work in configurations to build knowledge of whether they form necessary and/or sufficient conditions of the outcomes (such as health outcomes or health equity) we are interested in. This is done by calibrating causal factors in the cases as 'fuzzy sets' (on a scale between 0 and 1, with 0 being fully out of the set, and 1 being fully in the set, but 0.5 being indeterminate), and then exploring the set-theoretical relations between the causal factors and outcomes. Fuzzy sets are hybrid measures which combine quantitative (differences within kind) with qualitative (differences between kinds) measures. In exploring relationships, we look for necessary and/or sufficient conditions.

Necessary conditions are those where, when we consider an outcome, there seem to be a cause or causes consistently associated with it. So if countries with strong health outcomes consistently have low GINI coefficients, then there are grounds for claiming that GINI coefficients are a necessary condition for achieving strong health outcomes. In set-theoretical logic the outcome (strong health outcomes) is a subset of the necessary condition (low GINI coefficient). However, just because there seems to be a necessary condition, that does not mean the condition cannot lead to other outcomes as well. If a low GINI coefficient is a necessary condition for good health outcomes, that does not mean it cannot lead to other outcomes as well, such as perhaps health equity.

To find a sufficient condition, in contrast, the starting point is the causal conditions (rather than the outcomes), and then we look to see which outcomes are also consistently present. In set-theoretical terms the condition is a subset of the outcome, and finding a sufficient condition does not preclude an outcome from being achieved through other means than the one identified as well.

Individual sufficient conditions are fairly rare in social science – they tend to occur in configurations. So if a combination of high government funding and low voluntary health insurance was consistent with good access to healthcare, then that combination of factors would be a combined sufficient condition. However, there may be other ways of achieving good health access as well – finding a sufficient condition (or combination of conditions) does not mean that there are no other ways of also achieving the outcome we are interested in.

A strong interpretation of sufficient conditions (the 'veristic' approach (Ragin, 2000, 2008)) requires them always to be present in relation to the outcome being investigated, however Ragin's work has shown how to assess both necessary and sufficient conditions by assessing their set-theoretical consistency and coverage instead (Ragin, 2008). The book makes extensive use of those measures as, in dealing with the real world, there are always likely to be measurement errors, and because models of the world can never be entirely complete. To continue with the earlier example, it might be that a combination of high government funding and low voluntary health insurance is sufficient for good access to care, but it is unrealistic to expect those two conditions to achieve that outcome in every single case. Instead, Ragin's measures apply clear thresholds beyond which cases can be regarded as having necessary and sufficient conditions, and this allows 'deviant' cases to be identified and treated as a valuable source of learning to be explored in more detail to try and learn the reasons why what works for other countries does not appear to work in particular contexts or settings.

Where a country has a set of causal conditions which in other countries consistently lead to a particular outcome, but do not in that particular country, then this case is 'deviant for consistency'. It is also possible that cases can achieve a particular outcome (such as good access) while having a configuration of causal factors that do not suggest, when compared to other countries, that should happen. In Chapter 2, for example, this happens with social determinants and health outcomes for Australia. In these circumstances, it is again important to look harder at the case to explain what is going on, as that case is 'deviant for coverage'.

Having explained the method, then its application can now be outlined.

First, each outcome (social determinants, health funding and so on) was reviewed to find candidates which could be causal factors, and empirical measures for the chosen factors were sought. The best-fitting outcome measures for each chapter were then chosen. The measures were then compiled for each country, bringing together OECD and Commonwealth Fund data sources. The raw data for these measures and outcomes appear earlier in the chapter.

Second, initial expectations were generated about which countries were likely to fall into the 'in' and 'out' sets for each causal factor and each outcome. For example, the UK is generally regarded as having a health system which is, in international terms, not well funded, whereas the US is well known to have very high levels of funding.

Third, these initial expectations were compared to a mixture of graphical representations of the individual datasets, to explore the groupings of the countries into high or low sets. These results were then compared to cluster analysis for each of the factors, in order to make a final decision about where the 'out', 'crossover (between in and out)', and 'in' thresholds for each dataset were (this calibration process is shown in detail for each factor in the book's Appendix).

Fourth, each factor and outcome was given a calibrated set membership (between 0 and 1) along a curve between 0 representing non-membership, and 1 representing full membership (the full details of this are in the book's Appendix).

Once all the data had been calibrated, necessary relationships for each analysis (social determinants, health funding, spending, COVID) were identified according to measures of their consistency and relevance (coverage), but also their substantive relevance in relation to existing theory and research. The next stage is the construction of truth tables, which show all possible combinations of causal factors and outcomes, with counterfactual rows (where no empirical data were present) excluded from the analysis as they contain combinations of factors which were not technically possible. Truth table rows which achieved a high consistency measure in relation to the outcome measure were then identified, going back and forth between data and cases to validate those rows as strongly as possible.

Next, theoretical expectations for the data were generated, based on existing research and the findings for necessary conditions. These were incorporated into the generation of the sufficient intermediate solution (see later). Finally, at least three sufficient solutions were generated to explore the impact of making different assumptions about counterfactuals on the results; the parsimonious solution (taking all counterfactuals into account), the intermediate solution (taking only counterfactuals in line with theoretical expectations into account), and the conservative solution (taking no counterfactuals into account).

In general, and in line with enhanced standard analysis, the intermediate solution is the one presented in the findings sections that follow, but where the other solutions diverge to a significant degree, the implications of that divergence are explored.

The book therefore uses QCA to generate rigorous comparisons for the data in each chapter, generating solutions which allow us to compare our theoretical expectations to the results generated from the analysis, and so better understand the dynamics of health systems as a result. QCA therefore forms the backbone of the book, but its solutions require extensive interpretation, which forms the basis of the discussion and case-based analysis as a means of further and better understanding health systems.

Case studies

The book, as well as exploring data across cases, also needs to outline the relevant factors of the health systems it includes. This process will begin by outlining the health systems of Norway, Sweden and the Netherlands – three countries which, as the book develops, will be seen to consistently appear in high outcome solutions. Outlining these three cases early, then, gives some detail on countries which appear to do comparatively well in the dataset, and against which other countries can be compared as the book develops. The case studies were developed by combining data from a range of sources including the excellent Commonwealth Fund country profiles,[1] along with data from Johnson et al's extraordinary book (Johnson et al, 2017) and Boslaugh's reference guide (Boslaugh, 2013) as well as from national government websites. The decision was taken not to embed huge numbers of citations into the case study text to facilitate reading, especially when the data are mostly factual and can easily be found through the sources discussed earlier (and others). In each case study, the causal factor data for the book is also embedded to contextualise the case studies and link them to the relevant chapters.

The case studies begin with Norway, followed by Sweden and then the Netherlands.

Norway

Norway has a universal healthcare system, funded primarily from general taxes and from payroll contributions shared by both employers and employees. The national government is responsible for providing healthcare with the goal of ensuring equal access regardless of ability to pay or geographical location – with the second being especially challenging given Norway's geography. National government also regulates the health service, organises funding and oversees care provision, as well as being responsible for speciality care, which it also provides through state-owned regional health authorities. Services are primarily organised at the municipality level, which organises primary care and long-term care, but with the latter not being included in universal health insurance.

Private health insurance also exists to allow quicker access to service, as well as a wider choice of private providers, but is taken by a small percentage of people only. The service is comprehensive, covering primary and ambulatory care, as well as hospital and mental health care. Some prescription drugs are covered, but patients make co-payments, subject to caps, on a range of services.

Health insurance is automatic for all residents and is funded primarily through general taxation and out-of-pocket payments. Taxation, in turn, comes from transfers from general and municipal taxes, but also from payroll contributions. Municipalities receive their funding from block grants from the government and municipal taxes (around half each), and municipals are strongly linked to their health services as they comprise just over half of their total budgets.

Out-of-pocket payments cover nearly 15 per cent of total health expenditure, with co-payments occurring for most outpatient care services. However, there are annual caps and some exemptions, such as those for older people, those with communicable conditions such as HIV/AIDS, and those with permanent illnesses.

In terms of its membership of fuzzy sets for health funding, Norway's fuzzy-set scores are as follows:

COUNTRY	GOV	HEALTHEXP	OOP	VOL
NOR	0.95	0.99	0.84	0.02

From this, Norway has among the highest funding of all the countries considered in the book from government and compulsory insurance, is one of the heaviest spenders on healthcare, and makes use of very little voluntary health insurance. Perhaps surprisingly though, Norway also scores highly for out-of-pocket expenditure compared to the other countries explored in the book.

Residents can go to a GP of their choice, and individual GPs are overwhelmingly self-employed. GPs must provide referrals for access to specialist services. Public hospitals provide specialist care, with fees being set by central government, and with the central Ministry of Health and Care Services setting the Regional Health Authority budget.

Municipalities are responsible for organising long-term care, with most receiving care at home. Most nursing homes are owned and funded by municipalities, and service eligibility is needs based and means tested. Cost sharing is generally very high.

In terms of its expenditures, Norway's fuzzy-set scores are as follows:

COUNTRY	HEALTHEXP	CUREREHAB	LONG	PREVENT
NOR	0.99	0.21	0.97	0.24

Norway is one of the highest spenders on healthcare (as noted earlier), and in addition here it can be seen that it falls into the low sets for curative and rehabilitation expenditure, along with preventative care, but is a comparatively high spender on long-term care.

In relation to its social determinants, Norway has very low levels of income inequality and has low behavioural factors (smoking and drinking) compared to the other countries here. However, it also has higher numbers than we might expect of people with pre-secondary education only. This last factor is a key element of the social determinants of health, and we will explore whether it undermines the other factors which might be more favourable – such as low income inequality, low behavioural factors and high health expenditures.

COUNTRY	GINI	BEHAV	EDUC	HEALTHEXP
NOR	0.01	0.07	0.66	0.99

Sweden

Sweden has a health system which is universal, and in broad terms nationally regulated and locally administered. Health policy is set by the Ministry of Health and Social Affairs, with regions financing and delivering health services. Municipalities deliver social care. The health system is funded from regional and municipal taxation, supplemented by grants from central government, but with co-payments for primary care and hospital visits. Healthcare access is a citizenship right, with all legal residents being covered. Care is in every sense comprehensive, covering inpatient, outpatient, dental, mental health, long-term care, and prescription drugs. Sweden does not have a defined care package, with responsibility for care depending on regional governments, which vary in their provision of services to some degree across the country. Out-of-pocket payments make up around 15 per cent of all health expenditures, with regions setting co-payment rates, and so leading to some variation across the country. There are fees per service, but with maximum costs per year set for specialist consultations, hospital visits and prescription drugs. Private health insurance exists and is used to give improved access to specialists in the private health sector, but is taken out by very few people.

Healthcare is based around three principles – human dignity (equal entitlement to care regardless of status); need and solidarity (those with the greatest need have priority of access to care); cost-effectiveness (based on improvement in health and quality of life from treatment).

Sweden's health system is overwhelmingly funded from the public purse, with most expenditures coming from regions, where healthcare is their primary area of expenditure, and is funded by proportional income taxes.

Sweden's fuzzy-set scores for funding are as follows:

COUNTRY	GOV	HEALTHEXP	OOP	VOL
SWE	0.93	0.81	0.66	0.03

In terms of health funding, then, Sweden is very similar to Norway, scoring high in terms of overall health expenditure (although not as high as Norway), very high in terms of government and compulsory health insurance, and very low in terms of voluntary health insurance. Similarly, to Norway as well, Sweden also has higher out-of-pocket funding than we might have anticipated given its reputation as an archetypally social democratic nation.

GPs are usually the first point of contact for patients, but do not really fulfil a gatekeeper function as people can access other healthcare professionals directly should they so wish. The public nature of provision and funding makes the service highly integrated, but with regional and municipal governments having to ensure that collaboration between medical treatments and nursing and rehabilitation, respectively, is coordinated to avoid patients falling between the two levels of government.

Long-term care is financed through the municipalities and funded through taxation. Older adults and the disabled have a maximum co-payment of around $200 per month. Sweden's health expenditure fuzzy-set scores are as follows:

COUNTRY	HEALTHEXP	CUREREHAB	LONG	PREVENT
SWE	0.81	0.37	0.94	0.68

Again, there are strong similarities to Norway in terms of overall health expenditure, curative and rehabilitative expenditure levels (comparatively low) and long-term expenditure (very high). Preventative health expenditure in Sweden is relatively high, but lower in Norway.

In terms of its social determinants fuzzy-set scores, Sweden is as follows:

COUNTRY	GINI	BEHAV	EDUC	HEALTHEXP
SWE	0.06	0.06	0.69	0.81

Again, similarly to Norway, Sweden has very low income inequality, and very low behavioural (smoking and drinking factors), but higher numbers of people with pre-comprehensive levels of education only.

The Netherlands

The Netherlands has a universal health system which is based on private insurance. All residents are required to purchase health insurance from private insurers, with the private insurers required to accept all applicants. The uninsured are fined, and their premiums may be charged directly against their income, although people who object to insurance on a conscientious basis can opt to make mandatory payments into a health savings account instead. In practice only a very small number of people (around 0.2 per cent of the population) are uninsured. As health insurance is statutory, the funding of the system is categorised as coming through 'government or compulsory' sources, with insurance premiums being topped up by tax revenues and government grants. National legislation recognised access to health as being a right, including access to essential medicines.

Public funding is made up of earmarked payroll taxes from employers and employees, general taxation, insurance premiums, and co-payment. Statutory health insurance is financed through an annual income tax of around 7 per cent of income, and insurers have premiums that apply across all their enrolees, regardless of their age or health status. Income taxes and government grants are collected into a central health insurance fund and redistributed among insurers through a risk-adjusted capitation formula. In addition, over 80 per cent of people take out supplementary voluntary insurance to cover services not covered by statutory insurance, including dental care, eyeglasses, and contraceptives, and which also reduces co-payments for non-formulary medicines.

Out-of-pocket spending comes through a mandatory deductible of around $500, and an additional voluntary deductible of around $650 is available to reduce monthly premiums. People pay the full cost of specialty and hospital care up to the value of the deductible. Some services, including physiotherapy and some pharmaceuticals, may require additional co-payments even after the deductible is met. The government offers means-tested subsidies to help cover insurance premiums for low-income people, with nearly a third of the population receiving these allowances, which are set on a sliding, means-tested scale. In terms of its funding, the Netherlands calibrated fuzzy-set scores are as follows:

COUNTRY	GOVCOMP	HEALTHEXP	OOP	VOLPC
NLD	0.85	0.76	0.31	0.49

From this, the Netherlands has high government and compulsory funding. However, it is relatively low for its out-of-pocket funding, and its voluntary health insurance falls just below the crossover threshold, and so falls into the lower set.

Long-term care is financed separately from statutory health insurance through a statutory insurance system for this type of care alone. Taxpayers contribute just under 10 per cent of their income up to a maximum of around $45,000. The care covers residential care, personal care, medical and nursing care, as well as medical aids and transport. Eligibility is based on clinical need alone. The Netherlands is one of the highest spenders on long-term care, second only to Norway in this sample. Long-term care is provided by non–profit organisations which are privately owned, and there is extensive use of person budgets to encourage patients to make choices about their care.

The Netherlands' fuzzy–set scores for health expenditures are as follows:

COUNTRY	HEALTHEXP	CUREREHAB	LONG	PREVENT
NLD	0.76	0.08	0.93	0.87

As such, the Netherlands is a high healthcare spender, but compared to other countries in this book, spends relatively little on curative and rehabilitative services. In contrast, it is a high spender on long–term care and preventative care.

The national government sets overall health policy, including the setting of priorities for the system, monitoring access, ensuring quality and controlling costs. Those covered receive a range of standard benefits to cover doctor and hospital costs, prescription drugs, and any home nursing or mental healthcare they might need. There are deductibles in place, with co–payments required on some services and drugs. Municipalities are responsible for preventative screenings and long–term outpatient services.

In terms of social determinants, the Netherlands' fuzzy–set scores are as follows:

COUNTRY	GINI	BEHAV	EDUC	HEALTHEXP
NLD	0.07	0.68	0.93	0.76

From this, the Netherlands has low income inequality, but its rates of smoking and drinking are relatively high. Equally, its levels of people with pre–comprehensive education only are very high. The Netherlands, then, presents interesting questions as to whether its low levels of income inequality are undermined by its high behavioural factors and its high numbers of people with relatively low education levels.

2

Social determinants

Introduction

When comparisons of different health outcomes are carried out, there is still often an assumption that the reasons for those differences must be due to the performance of the health services in those countries. Politicians and policymakers debate league tables of health outcomes as if the results are entirely dependent on what goes on in healthcare services, and plans are put in place to attempt to address what have been identified on problem areas (Greener, 2016). However, it may often be the case that the health outcomes differences between different countries may be due to factors *outside* of the direct control of healthcare services.

Healthcare services are undoubtedly important, and the book will explore how they are funded, and what the money is spent on, in Chapters 3 and 4. But however important healthcare is, our health depends on a range of other factors that fall outside the remit or control of healthcare organisations and institutions (Schrecker and Bambra, 2015).

In respect of our own lives, we are fully aware that health services are not the only, or perhaps even the most important, factors in determining our health. Whether we can access health services (or not) when we are ill or injured is clearly important. This will be especially the case where people have a serious injury or life-threatening illness, but is also the case for the millions of people with long-term health problems that may require medications or medical devices, as in the case of diabetes or asthma.

At the same time, there are a range of factors which are likely to affect our health, but which generally fall outside of the control or remit of most health services. These factors are often referred to as the 'social determinants' of health, and go from those that might come most quickly to mind, such as the levels of smoking and drinking, and other activities we have come to associate with poor health outcomes, as well as education levels and the quality of housing available. However, there may also be much larger social factors, such as levels of inequality, which those taking a more large-scale, social determinants approach suggest are extremely important.

Large-scale social determinants such as inequality or poverty are especially important because they intersect across a range of factors to produce systematic effects: the poorest people tend to smoke more than those with higher incomes, may have access to only lower-quality housing and are likely to have successfully completed less education (Mullainathan and Shafir, 2013). The social determinants of health can be separated analytically, but are likely to cluster and combine in particular ways so that poor health outcomes especially are linked to a combination of different factors. This intersectionality seems to be especially the case for people in some minority groupings (Ragin and Fiss, 2016) to the extent that some writers have come close to claiming that racial differences underlie differences in societal outcomes (Hernstein and Murray, 1996), when this seems to confuse cause and effect. Some social groups face intersectional disadvantages, but the colour of people's skin or ethnicity does not determine this.

The next section explores existing research on the social determinants of health, explaining which causal factors will be considered, and with the section after that outlining the data that will be used.

Social determinants of health

Even once the importance of the social determinants of health has been accepted, establishing exactly which factors should be taken into account in a comparative study of health systems is not a straightforward task.

The American Public Health Association, for example, published a graph on life expectancy, corresponding to the 2014 version of the Commonwealth Fund report (Figure 2.1).

Figure 2.1 shows some degree of variation between countries (although the Y axis is quite compressed), with Australia having the highest life expectancy for the countries included here, and the US the lowest. The reasons given in the report for the US's relatively poor performance give one factor which is at least related to health services (poor birth outcomes), but the rest cover a range of social factors, such as injuries and homicides, prevalence of heart disease, obesity and diabetes, disability, adolescent pregnancy and sexually transmitted disease rates, HIV and AIDS prevalence and drug-related deaths. These factors are, in turn, often interrelated and clustered in relation to inequalities of wealth and ethnicity.

Studies which 'zoom out' and look at changes in life expectancy over the last 30 years, comparing nations in terms of their similarities and differences, can help to provide common factors which appear

Figure 2.1: Life expectancy at birth, 2014

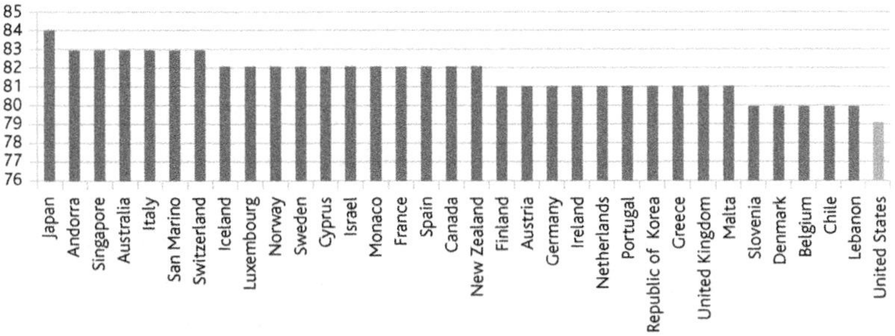

From America's Health Rankings, ©2021 United Health Foundation, https://www.apha.org/
topics-and-issues/health-rankings

to help to account for those changes. There is a body of work which attributes a large role in improvements in health outcomes to increases in overall health expenditures (Deaton, 2015). In addition to this, work by the OECD (2017), as well as confirming the insight about health expenditures and improved life expectancy, also points to declining drinking and smoking rates, and a decline in the proportion of people at the lowest education levels, as being statistically linked as well. As such, the OECD work incorporates a mix of spending and social factors.

All these factors make a great deal of sense in terms of existing theory and research being able to explain why they should be important causes for better or worse health outcomes. Higher expenditure on health systems could improve access to high-quality care, improve health equity and make sure the best treatments are available. Higher health expenditures may also improve health education and put in place better strategies for preventative care. Declining rates of smoking and drinking (which is the case for just about all developed nations) should reduce the risk factors associated with those behaviours. If people are better educated, they should be able to make better choices about their health, as well as potentially having access to better work and life opportunities. As well as this, there is clear evidence that slowing rises in life expectancy (or even reductions) are linked to rises in 'deaths of despair' (Case and Deaton, 2020), which fall disproportionately on those with lower levels of education only.

These factors – health expenditure, smoking and drinking, and education – do not tell the whole story. It is becoming clear that health outcomes are subject to a 'gap' (Marmot, 2015) between the richest and poorest within countries' own borders, but also between different countries. Marmot and other writers (Wilkinson and Pickett,

2010) have developed theories about how this gap causes differences in health outcomes based on what Marmot calls 'status syndrome' (Marmot, 2012) and which has strong parallels to what Wilkinson and Pickett refer to as the 'inner level' (Wilkinson and Pickett, 2018). Here differences in income and wealth are linked to disadvantaged people having a smaller 'locus of control' over their lives, which the researchers associate with increased stress and a range of adverse social factors such as increased illness. However, increased inequalities also lead, in the view of these researchers, to a decrease in trust between social groups and increases in a range of 'social ills', including more risky health behaviours and crime. In this view, inequality is important not only because some groups will be affected most by 'status anxiety' and suffer poorer health outcomes, but also because more unequal societies become more stressful for everyone living in them – including those who have high levels of income and wealth – because of the decline in trust and increase in crime. This point is emphasised in the American Public Health Association's work with which this section begins, which states 'it's not just low-income and minority groups driving the trend. It's true across all ages and incomes. In the U.S., even if you are white, high income, well-educated and have good insurance, you appear to be in worse health than your peers in other developed countries.'[1]

In addition to inequality, writers such as Marmot, in common with the OECD, point to the importance of education, with special concern for people with low levels (generally pre-secondary) of education only. There is again a credible argument here. If people have low levels of education, they are likely to have fewer opportunities to achieve meaningful work, so having a reduced locus of control over their lives, as well as being more likely to be in lower-income work (or depending on benefits), and living in poorer-quality housing. Lower levels of education may also make navigating through society more stressful, creating the potential to have a reduced capacity for leading healthier lifestyles (Mullainathan and Shafir, 2013) and so the greater possibility of engaging in less healthy behaviours. As noted earlier, health disadvantages tend to cluster, with lower levels of education acting, in a similar way to ethnicity, as a point at which those clusters congregate. Minority groups in society may also face intersectional disadvantages, with clusters of low income, poor housing, access to poorer schools and less meaningful work, which combine to lead to poorer health outcomes (Bambra, 2011, 2017).

Looking across the factors identified here, then, different theories of the social determinants of health begin to surface. The first is perhaps the simplest – that overall levels of health expenditures are strongly linked to health outcomes, at least at the national level. This very simple view is barely a theory of the social determinants of health as it does not include factors which would commonly be regarded as 'social', such as inequality or education. However, it is certainly worth including health expenditures as a key factor which might help us in exploring differences between countries. From the OECD life expectancy research presented earlier, an extended version of the health expenditure theory can come through including risk factors such as smoking and drinking, and also education levels, as being important.

On the other hand, Marmot and a range of social determinants researchers seem to take a different approach, putting inequality at the heart of their analyses and linking income inequality especially (wealth inequality is very difficult to measure comparatively) to a range of health and other social problems. In Marmot's work there are also regular references to educational levels, as well as to the importance of looking at inequalities in the intersectional way described earlier. It is also clear that other factors, such as ethnicity, are important in comparing health systems. The challenge here is that comparative measures of minority groups are extremely difficult to construct. As such, although the book would ideally incorporate ethnicity, it will not be included here.

It is important to emphasise that these sets of factors (health expenditure, smoking and drinking rates, education on the one hand, and inequality and education on the other) are not necessarily mutually exclusive – it is quite possible that higher levels of health expenditure can exist alongside either high or low levels of inequality, for example, to produce different health outcomes. However, there is relatively little work exploring these determinants of health in such an intersectional and conjunctional way. Equally, it may well be possible to achieve good health outcomes through a number of different combinations of the factors outlined earlier, and it is important to consider the possibility of this factor, which is called 'equifinality'.

Considering the social determinants of health in an intersectional way means considering how these factors combine in countries with higher health outcomes, and whether some of the factors, although their effect has been demonstrated in existing research, might prove to be less significant towards that goal. Looking at the factors in this way might suggest which are the most urgent for policymakers to address.

This chapter explores this range of factors – health expenditure, levels of smoking, drinking and education, and income inequality in a conjunctional way, to explore the extent they explain differences in health outcomes, but also health equity, between nations.

This next section outlines the data used in this chapter's analysis, justifying the specific measures and giving a preliminary assessment of patterns in the data.

Because tobacco and alcohol consumption are factors which can be categorised as behavioural, they were combined into one behavioural factor. The behavioural factor therefore summarises health and smoking statistics across our countries, resulting in an index where the two factors are simply added together to generate an overall behavioural risk factor. The two factors are added together as this results in tobacco being about double-weighted compared to alcohol. This factor was then compared (in terms of results) to those derived from the separate factors, and it made little difference to the set-theoretical categorisation of countries, but did help simplify results a little. This combined behavioural factor is therefore included in the analysis below.

Having calibrated the data in line with the principles outlined in Chapter 1, and with the book's Appendix giving a more detailed account, the results were as shown in Table 2.1.

In turn, this can produce an initial clustering of the countries in which scores above 0.5 for a factor result in a 1, and scores below 0.5 with a 0, to show countries that are 'in' or 'out' of sets (scores of 0.5 would have be excluded as neither in or out of the fuzzy set). In this book most of the data being analysed have been measured in terms of causal factors and outcomes, where, in order to try and make results more interpretable, where the set name appears (such as GINI) it will

Table 2.1: Social determinants calibrated dataset

COUNTRY	GINI	BEHAV	EDUC	HEALTHEXP
AUS	0.68	0.28	0.85	0.30
CAN	0.28	0.23	0.04	0.33
FRA	0.11	0.97	0.90	0.24
GER	0.13	0.93	0.23	0.83
NLD	0.07	0.68	0.93	0.76
NZ	0.89	0.37	0.95	0.02
NOR	0.01	0.07	0.66	0.99
SWE	0.06	0.06	0.69	0.81
SWI	0.15	0.86	0.19	1.00
UK	0.91	0.70	0.82	0.08
US	0.99	0.12	0.06	1.00

Table 2.2: Country clustering for the social determinants of health

GINI	BEHAV	EDUC	HEALTHEXP	CASES
0	0	0	0	CAN
0	0	1	1	NOR, SWE
0	1	1	1	NLD
0	1	0	1	GER, SWI
0	1	1	0	FRA
1	0	0	1	US
1	0	1	0	AUS, NZ
1	1	1	0	UK

refer to the countries having scores measured as 'high' in value. Where the name appears with a ~ in front of it (as in ~GINI), it will refer to countries that are not in the high set. This is technically not quite the same thing as 'low', but in terms of shorthand and interpretability, that is how it will be referred to throughout the book, as the countries have a great deal in common, and the results need to be as understandable as possible. The results for social determinants can be summarised in Table 2.2.

Australia, New Zealand, the UK and the US fall into the set of countries with high income inequality, having 1 in the GINI column in Table 2.2. The countries with 0, in contrast, are not in the high set. From the research discussed earlier, countries which score 1 for their GINI measure might be expected to perform poorly in terms of health outcomes and health equity on the basis of that factor alone. As explained earlier, the link to health outcomes comes through the work of Marmot and is theorised in terms of a 'health gap' in which more unequal countries create greater status anxiety between people, and with that stress resulting in a loss of sense of autonomy and control over people's lives. This should leave the countries with low income inequality performing better in terms of those measures.

Looking more interjectionally, the behavioural index creates an interesting tension in relation to income inequality. Three of the countries with behavioural factors scored as 0 (so out of the high scoring set – Canada, Norway and Sweden) also have zero scores for inequality, but the Netherlands, France, Germany and Switzerland have high behavioural indexes (scores of 1) and income inequality scores of zero. These combinations raise the question of whether such differences might lead, in turn, to differences in health outcomes and health equity, or whether low levels of income inequality might be able to offset these higher levels of behavioural factors. It is also the case that three countries that have lower behavioural factors (Australia, New Zealand and the US) have high income inequality. What difference does that make?

The next column (EDUC) explores the levels of people with low levels of education – so lower numbers here suggest that a country has fewer people who might have poorer health outcomes. The countries with the lowest levels of secondary education only are Canada and the US, followed by Switzerland and Germany. Canada, then, appears to have low income inequality, low behavioural factors and low levels of people with pre-secondary education only – in terms of the first three factors it has the strongest possible 'fit' with an expectation of high health equity and high health outcomes. The US, in contrast, has high GINI, low behavioural factors and a very low level of people with pre-secondary education only. This combination of factors asks whether the relatively good behavioural and educational factors might be sufficient to offset its levels of income inequality – which are the highest of all the nations here. The combinations of factors for Germany and Switzerland ask a different question – whether the disadvantage of high levels of behavioural factors are enough to overcome the advantages of having a relatively low GINI and low levels of pre-secondary education only.

The final column covers health expenditure, which is the factor in common across all the analyses in the book. At the top end there is the US, which spends most in the world ($9892 per capita) and is an extreme outlier, and that means that Switzerland (the second-highest spender), Norway, Germany and the Netherlands are also categorised as very high spenders. The lowest spender in the sample is the UK at $4192 – less than half that of the US. The key question health expenditures raise in the context of this chapter is whether, in combination with other factors, the countries that spend the most also have the best outcomes of all kinds, or whether expenditure levels form patterns with other causal factors. In the case of the US, does its extraordinarily high level of expenditure, along with its strong behavioural and educational factors, offset its high income inequality? In the case of the UK, we might predict poor performance for both health outcomes and health equity as here it has a high GINI, high behavioural factors, high levels of people with pre-secondary education only, and the lowest health expenditure of all. Based on existing research, this seems like the worst possible combination of factors.

Directional expectations

In order to generate intermediate sufficient solutions, what is called 'directional expectations' need to be incorporated into the calculations. Directional expectations distinguish which counterfactual lines in the truth table – or patterns of causal factors which do not appear in the data – are included in the calculation of the intermediate sufficient solution term, with only those matching directional expectations being included. For health outcomes, and given the research discussed earlier, high health expenditure is supported in terms of most the research, and so there is a strong case for its inclusion. As low inequality appears at the forefront of work by Marmot and Wilkinson and Pickett, this term also has a strong case for inclusion. Finally, as there is overwhelming evidence in support of lower drinking and smoking, low behavioural factors seem supported by the existing research. Lower levels of pre-secondary education are not included as a directional expectation as the link to health outcomes is not as established in existing research as centrally as for the other factors. It is important to emphasise, however, that not being included as a directional expectation does not preclude lower levels of pre-secondary education from appearing in sufficient intermediate solutions should there be existing empirical support for the factor, and it may appear in either parsimonious or conservative solutions which are not affected by directional expectations.

For health equity, directional expectations were a little different. Existing research supports low levels of inequality and higher levels of health expenditure supporting health equity, with the former being linked to more equitable societies more generally, and the latter with the capacity of countries to afford to widen access to care. In addition, however, rather than behavioural factors, lower levels of pre-secondary education were included because of the link between education and health equity, with higher levels of education, in line with existing research, leading to lower levels of long-term risky health behaviours and an increased capacity to engage with public health messages.

The next section explores how these factors play out in terms of the results for health outcomes, before moving on to health equity. After that the discussion will consider the results in greater depth.

Results: high health outcomes

This section considers the combinations of social determinant factors which countries with high health outcomes (those scoring above 0.5 in the calibrated dataset) achieve. The full calibrated dataset for social

Table 2.3: Calibrated dataset for health outcomes

COUNTRY	GINI	BEHAV	EDUC	HEALTHEXP	HEALTH OUTCOMES
AUS	0.68	0.28	0.85	0.30	0.95
CAN	0.28	0.23	0.04	0.33	0.19
FRA	0.11	0.97	0.90	0.24	0.76
GER	0.13	0.93	0.23	0.83	0.32
NLD	0.07	0.68	0.93	0.76	0.54
NZ	0.89	0.37	0.95	0.02	0.38
NOR	0.01	0.07	0.66	0.99	0.89
SWE	0.06	0.06	0.69	0.81	0.94
SWI	0.15	0.86	0.19	1.00	0.83
UK	0.91	0.70	0.82	0.08	0.07
US	0.99	0.12	0.06	1.00	0.04

determinants is shown in Table 2.3, with the health outcomes measure in the column furthest to the right.

The first stage of analysis is to look for combinations of conditions which are necessary – which are found by considering the countries with outcome measures above 0.5, and seeing which causal factors (GINI, BEHAV, EDUC, HEALTHEXP) or combinations of causal factors are consistently present or absent in relation to that outcome measure.

To be a necessary condition there are two hurdles. The first is statistical. If necessary conditions have high consistency in relation to the outcome (using 0.8 as an initial measure), and explain a high proportion of the outcome, then there is a case for considering them necessary. As such, necessary conditions have to be highly consistent with the outcome, but also 'relevant' to it (Ragin, 2008, p 62). A minimum requirement of 0.6 relevancy was set, in line with the examples given by Dusa (2018). The second hurdle is to consider the results obtained statistically, and to make sure they are also substantively important – that they help us understand the outcome in terms of existing theory or research.

For high health outcomes, low income inequality (~GINI) was found to be a necessary condition, with a consistency of 0.84 and a relevance of 0.71. The consistency level is a little lower than the 0.9 generally used in examples by Dusa (2018), but also appears in both pathways to sufficient solutions in the results below, and is strongly supported in existing research, so it makes sense to include ~GINI as necessary for high health outcomes, given the social determinants factors included here.

This is an important first finding. In the solutions that follow it is necessary, in terms of the social determinants of health, for a country to have low income inequality to achieve high health outcomes. Looking across the cases in the dataset presented earlier, this finding applies to all but one of the countries (France, the Netherlands, Norway, Sweden and Switzerland) with health outcome scores calibrated greater than 0.5, with Australia as the exception (which helps explain why the consistency score is 0.84 rather than being even closer to 1.0). However, just because ~GINI is a necessary condition, that does not mean that all ~GINI countries have high health outcomes, (as with Canada and Germany) – this stage of analysis is identifying necessary, not sufficient, factors.

To find causal factors which consistently lead to high health outcomes a sufficient solution has to be calculated. The first stage of this is to construct a truth table. This requires a consistency threshold to be set, and here a threshold of 0.785 was utilised, which is a little below the ideal 0.8 benchmark, but which allowed the inclusion of Switzerland, albeit at the expense also of bringing in Germany, which was a case deviant for consistency. However, the sufficient solution utilising the higher consistency threshold will also be outlined later.

This resulted in the truth table (Table 2.4).

Table 2.4 takes a little explanation.

The first four columns are the fuzzy-set scores derived earlier (and in the book's Appendix in more detail), but expressed here in terms of the single combination which achieves a combined score of over 0.5. For Canada, the first row, this is a combination of low BEHAV, low GINI, low EDUC and low HEALTH EXP. This would be expressed

Table 2.4: Truth table for social determinants and high health outcomes

BEHAV	GINI	EDUC	HEALTH EXP	OUT	CONSISTENCY	PRI	CASES
0	0	0	0	0	0.617	0.314	CAN
0	0	1	1	1	0.992	0.987	NOR, SWE
0	1	0	1	0	0.471	0.101	US
0	1	1	0	0	0.740	0.562	AUS, NZ
1	0	0	1	1	0.786	0.595	GER, SWI
1	0	1	0	1	0.980	0.954	FRA
1	0	1	1	1	0.916	0.667	NLD
1	1	1	0	0	0.638	0.266	UK

as ~BEHAV★~GINI★~EDUC★~HEALTH EXP. In that formula, ★ means AND. A little confusingly, in fuzzy-set theory, + means OR. Where the ★ operator appears, the lowest score of the two factors is used (the weakest link), and where the + operator appears, the higher of the two (the strongest link). Where a factor appears with nothing in front of it (as in GINI) it is referring to the high set (above 0.5) of calibrated scores, but where a ~ appears in front of the name (as in ~GINI) it is referring to the negative set (below 0.5) of scores – the values which are not in the high set.

The OUT column shows whether the combination of factors was included in the solution calculation or not, and is dependent on the consistency threshold used to calculate the truth table, with the individual row consistency levels in the next column (CONSISTENCY). A general rule of thumb across the QCA methods books is to take a consistency of 0.8, but there is some room for judgement. Here the choice was between taking a consistency of 0.8, which would also produce the same solution up to a consistency level of 0.915 (with the Netherlands having a consistency of 0.916), or reducing consistency to 0.785 to include the cases of Germany and Switzerland. The solution that follows was calculated with a truth table of consistency of 0.785, but will also explain what difference this choice makes in the generation of the solution.

Finally, the column PRI stands for 'proportional reduction in inconsistency' and is an additional measure of consistency. The key thing, in brief, is that where there is a truth table line with a high consistency score but a low PRI score, there is the possibility of cases appearing as being included in both the solution for the high (here high health outcomes) and low sets, and that is something which needs to be avoided.

With a consistency threshold of 0.785 and directional expectations that high health outcomes would result from low behavioural factors, low income inequality and high health expenditure (~BEHAV★~GINI★HEALTH EXP), the following intermediate sufficient solution was generated:

Solution	Consistency	PRI	Coverage	Unique coverage	Cases
~GINI*EDUC	0.867	0.788	0.612	0.319	FRA, NLD, NOR, SWE
BEHAV*~GINI*HEALTH EXP	0.778	0.564	0.442	0.149	GER, NLD, SWI
Overall solution consistency 0.798, coverage 0.761					

The intermediate sufficient solution suggests two pathways to achieving high health outcomes. Again, some explanation of the numbers is needed.

The consistency of the solution is assessed by taking the sum of the minimum of the causal factors (in the first solution pathway ~GINI*EDUC) and the outcome (high health outcomes), and dividing by the sum of the solution pathway. Where all the causal factors scores are equal to or lower than the outcome scores, then the solution consistency is 1.0, and the causal factors are a subset of the outcome measure – indicating a sufficient set-theoretical relationship between the two. So the nearer to 1.0, the more consistent the solution, but where the measure drops below 0.5, then this indicates that our causal factor scores are higher than the outcome measures, and that there is low consistency (Ragin, 2008, p 52). The PRI score gives us an additional measure of consistency, and a low PRI score (below 0.4) would give reason for concern. 'Coverage' measures how much of the outcome measure the particular combination of causal factors explains, and unique coverage is a measure of how much of the outcome measure the combination of causal factors covers which is not covered by other solution pathways.

Solution terms with high consistency, high coverage and the highest unique coverage scores have strong empirical support, but it is also necessary to look to see which cases the solution terms cover, and whether the solution terms make substantive sense.

The first solution pathway is a combination of low income inequality and higher levels of people with pre-secondary education only. The first of these two factors fits with existing research, and with our calculation of ~GINI as a necessary condition, but the second is rather more surprising. This solution covers the cases of France, the Netherlands, Norway and Sweden.

The second solution pathway, which is removed if the consistency threshold is increased to 0.786, is a combination of low income inequality (as with the first pathway, and in line with it being a necessary condition), but combined with high health expenditure, and high behavioural factors. Two of these three factors (low GINI and high health expenditure) fit with existing research, so here the surprising factor is that of high behavioural factors.

If the truth table consistency level is raised above 0.786, indeed as high as 0.91, then the solution is the first pathway of the solution only. This increases the consistency of the overall solution to 0.867, but reduces its coverage to 0.612 – the same numbers that are in the first solution pathway.

No theoretical model will perfectly capture reality, and that means that there are always likely to be 'deviant' cases. In the solution there are two of these cases, one which appears in the solution, but does not achieve high health outcomes (Germany), and one which achieved high health outcomes but does not appear in the solution (Australia).

In the second solution pathway, GER is included, but has a fuzzy-set score of 0.32 – so below the 0.5 threshold. It is therefore a deviant case for consistency. This means that although Germany has a pattern of causal factors (BEHAVE*~GINI*HEALTH EXP), which, in the Netherlands and Sweden, has a sufficient relationship to high health outcomes, in Germany they do not. It is therefore important to try and identify why this is and to consider what is different about the German case.

It is possible to remove Germany as a deviant case for consistency by raising the consistency threshold of the truth table to 0.786. However, because Germany is on the same truth table row as Switzerland, with the same pattern of social determinants (BEHAV*~GINI*~EDUC*HEALTHEXP), then this would result in Switzerland being excluded from the solution term. Switzerland then would become a case which is deviant for 'coverage' – or a country which is 'missing' from the solution.

One country is missing from the sufficient solution, namely Australia, which has very strong health outcomes, but does not appear in the solution because its patterns of causal factors (GINI*~BEHAV*EDUC*~HEALTH EXP), and which it has in common with New Zealand, is not consistent with high health outcomes (from our truth table it has a consistency score of 0.74). It is therefore important to try and work out what it is about Australia that means, despite its pattern of causal factors, it still achieves high health outcomes. The cases of both Germany and Australia will be revisited in the discussion section of this chapter.

The conservative version of the sufficient solution is more complex than the intermediate one presented earlier, as it does not include counterfactual rows – the patterns of causes for which there are no empirical data. In the conservative solution, the second solution pathway is identical, but the first is split into two subsets, both of which have ~GINI*EDUC in common. As such, the intermediate solution pathways seem fairly robust.

The parsimonious solution has ~GINI*EDUC in common with the solution, but simplifies the second pathway to BEHAV*~GINI. These solution terms then appear not to change the understanding of the sufficient solutions in a significant way.

The book will return to a discussion of these findings later in the chapter. However, it now moves on to explore the combinations of social determinants factors which have a necessary or sufficient relationship to high health equity.

Results: high health equity

The calibrated data for the social determinants of health in relation to health equity are shown in Table 2.5.

From Table 2.5, the countries with high health equity are Germany, the Netherlands, Norway, Sweden, Switzerland and the UK. The first task, as with high health outcomes, is to examine whether necessary conditions are in place.

For high health equity, the necessary condition of low GINI (~GINI) was considered as a possible candidate, and among the high equity countries Germany, the Netherlands, Norway, Sweden and Switzerland have this term in common, but the UK does not. As such, the UK prevents ~GINI from meeting the statistical threshold for being considered. The highest scoring necessary condition was a combination of low GINI OR high behavioural factors (~GINI + BEHAV). Whereas there is research supporting low GINI, high behavioural factors are not supported by existing work, and the relevance score of 0.55 is at the low end of empirical support. As such, no factor or combination of factors was included as a necessary condition for high health equity.

Table 2.5: Calibrated dataset for social determinants and high health equity

COUNTRY	GINI	BEHAV	EDUC	HEALTHEXP	EQUITY
AUS	0.68	0.28	0.85	0.30	0.36
CAN	0.28	0.23	0.04	0.33	0.16
FRA	0.11	0.97	0.90	0.24	0.10
GER	0.13	0.93	0.23	0.83	0.51
NLD	0.07	0.68	0.93	0.76	0.87
NZ	0.89	0.37	0.95	0.02	0.27
NOR	0.01	0.07	0.66	0.99	0.64
SWE	0.06	0.06	0.69	0.81	0.83
SWI	0.15	0.86	0.19	1.00	0.81
UK	0.91	0.70	0.82	0.08	0.98
US	0.99	0.12	0.06	1.00	0.02

Table 2.6: Truth table for social determinants and high health equity

BEHAV	GINI	EDUC	HEALTHEXP	OUT	CONSISTENCY	PRI	CASES
0	0	0	0	0	0.619	0.151	CAN
0	0	1	1	1	0.992	0.982	NOR, SWE
0	1	0	1	0	0.456	0.063	US
0	1	1	0	0	0.637	0.290	AUS, NZ
1	0	0	1	1	0.859	0.222	FRA
1	0	1	1	1	0.927	0.816	NLD
1	1	1	0	1	0.983	0.863	UK

The truth table (Table 2.6) was produced with a consistency of 0.8, but the same results appear up to a consistency threshold of 0.858, which is well above the 0.8 benchmark.

Table 2.6, as it is based on the same pattern of causal factors as was used for high health outcomes, has the same pattern for the first four columns. However, the OUT column, which determines whether the truth table row is included in the calculation for sufficiency, is different, as are the consistency and PRI scores, as these results are based on the health equity outcome (rather than the health outcome measure in Table 2.4).

The intermediate sufficient solution was based on directional expectations of low income inequality, high health expenditure and low levels of pre-secondary education. These three factors are the most strongly empirically supported in relation to health equity, with smoking and drinking linked more to outcomes and so not being included as an expectation, although this does not exclude them from being included should there be empirical support in the data, and directional expectations make no difference to the calculation of conservative or parsimonious solutions.

The intermediate sufficient solution was as follows:

Solution	Consistency	PRI	Coverage	Unique coverage	Case
BEHAV*GINI	0.877	0.714	0.349	0.159	UK
~GINI*HEALTHEXP	0.805	0.689	0.756	0.565	GER, NLD, NOR, SWE, SWI

Solution consistency 0.807, coverage 0.914

There are two solution pathways to high equity.

The first applies to the UK only and is a combination of high behavioural factors and high GINI. The review of existing research discussed earlier suggested that neither of these factors, either in themselves or in combination, would lead to good health equity. What this solution suggests is that social determinants seem unlikely to be playing a significant role as causal factors in contributing towards equity for the UK – that its high equity score is due to other factors. Possible reasons for the UK's high health equity score will be picked up in the discussion section.

The second solution pathway is much more aligned with our theoretical expectations and existing research, combining a low GINI with high health expenditure, and covers the cases of Norway, Sweden, Germany, Switzerland and the Netherlands. This pathway has very high coverage, and by far the highest unique coverage, suggesting it is both empirically and theoretically important.

The sufficient solution here has no cases which are deviant for consistency or coverage, so that all of the countries included in the solution have a high health equity score, and there are no countries which achieve a high health equity score that are missing from the solution. The lack of deviant cases adds further credibility to the solution.

The parsimonious solution is identical to the intermediate one presented previously. The conservative solution, which takes account of no counterfactuals, splits the second solution pathway into two subsets which are more complex, one of which adds high behavioural factors (to the existing solution terms) to cover Germany, Switzerland and the Netherlands, and the second of which adds high levels of pre-secondary education (to the existing solution terms) to cover Norway, Sweden and the Netherlands. Each of these solutions is less theoretically persuasive than the one in the previous intermediate solution, as each includes a factor which strong existing research would suggest is not linked to high health equity. As such, the intermediate solution terms appear the most strongly supported by existing research.

Results: high health equity and health outcomes

Finally, in terms of results, this chapter considers patterns of social determinant causal factors that lead to both high equity and high health outcomes. To accomplish this in set-theoretical logic, a logical AND calculation was performed on the two sets of outcome measures, which has the effective result of taking the lower score of the two. This

Table 2.7: Calibrated data for social determinants and high equity AND health outcomes

COUNTRY	GINI	BEHAV	EDUC	HEALTHEXP	EQUITY AND HEALTH OUTCOMES
AUS	0.68	0.28	0.85	0.30	0.36
CAN	0.28	0.23	0.04	0.33	0.16
FRA	0.11	0.97	0.90	0.24	0.10
GER	0.13	0.93	0.23	0.83	0.32
NLD	0.07	0.68	0.93	0.76	0.54
NZ	0.89	0.37	0.95	0.02	0.27
NOR	0.01	0.07	0.66	0.99	0.64
SWE	0.06	0.06	0.69	0.81	0.83
SWI	0.15	0.86	0.19	1.00	0.81
UK	0.91	0.70	0.82	0.08	0.07
US	0.99	0.12	0.06	1.00	0.02

is a demanding measure as it means the weakest of the two results is taken forward as the outcome score. That calculation resulted in the calibrated data shown in Table 2.7.

The first step is to see if necessary conditions are present in these data. A search revealed that ~GINI*HEALTHEXP had a consistency of 0.92 and a relevance of 0.8, so clearly met the empirical threshold. From Table 2.7, the Netherlands, Norway, Sweden and Switzerland have scores above 0.5 for EQUITY AND HEALTH OUTCOME, and in each case that they have a score below 0.5 for GINI and a score above 0.5 for health expenditure (~GINI*HEALTHEXP), and as such these meet the statistical requirement for being necessary conditions for the achievement of both high equity and health outcomes. More importantly, this combination of factors is also entirely in line with existing theory – a low GINI coefficient is consistent with the claims made by Marmot (and others) in terms of both health outcomes, and achieving strong health outcomes for a population is at least partially dependent on there being the necessary health resources available.

The truth table (Table 2.8) was calculated with a consistency threshold of 0.8, but with the same result being generated up to 0.842, so above the 0.8 benchmark.

From Table 2.8, there are two rows included in the solution term – those with Norway and Sweden, and further down, the Netherlands. Although Switzerland has a score above 0.5 for health equity and

Table 2.8: Truth table for social determinants and high health equity AND health outcomes

BEHAV	GINI	EDUC	HEALTHEXP	OUT	CONSISTENCY	PRI	CASES
0	0	0	0	0	0.599	0.032	CAN
0	0	1	1	1	0.984	0.954	NOR, SWE
0	1	0	1	0	0.446	0.000	US
0	1	1	0	0	0.514	0.000	AUS, NZ
1	0	0	1	0	0.771	0.530	GER, SWI
1	0	1	0	0	0.604	0.000	FRA
1	0	1	1	1	0.843	0.198	NLD
1	1	1	0	0	0.577	0.000	UK

health outcomes, that country appears on the same truth table row as Germany, and so achieves a consistency score of 0.771, and so is not included in the calculation of the sufficient solution that follows (although the result if consistency is lowered will be explained).

The intermediate sufficient solution was calculated with directional expectations of low GINI and high current expenditure, given the empirical support for those factors in the previous results, as well as with existing research. The result was as follows:

Solution	Consistency	PRI	Coverage	Cases
~GINI*EDUC*HEALTHEXP	0.876	0.688	0.685	NLD, NOR, SWE

The intermediate sufficient solution for high health equity and outcomes is a three term configuration combining low GINI, high levels of pre-secondary education only and high health expenditure. The solution covers Norway, Sweden and the Netherlands.

The conservative and parsimonious solutions, in this case, are identical to the intermediate one.

As noted earlier, the solution here has Switzerland deviant for coverage. If the truth table consistency threshold is lowered to 0.77, this retains the earlier solution pathway, but adds an additional solution pathway compromised of high behavioural factors, low GINI and high health expenditure, which covers Germany, Switzerland and the Netherlands, but which introduces Germany as a case deviant for consistency.

As such, there are two credible solutions, one of which has a case deviant for coverage (Switzerland) and one a case deviant for consistency (Germany). Given the higher consistency and parsimony of the first solution, it seems reasonable to prefer that intermediate solution.

With a necessary condition of ~GINI*HEALTHEXP, the combination of these two factors seems crucial to understanding success for high health equity and health outcomes, and indeed these solution terms appear in the pathway in the solution(combined with higher levels of low education, so forming a superset of that solution term). Both these factors will therefore be carried forward to Chapter 6 as the most important in terms of social determinants.

Discussion of results

In terms of health outcomes, there are three broad theories with which to compare our results.

The first is simply one around health expenditure: do the countries that spend the most achieve the best health outcomes? The second is around income inequality and education: are the best health outcomes in the countries with the lowest GINI coefficients and the lowest levels of people with low levels of education? The third is related to health behaviours: do countries with the lowest levels of health behaviours have the best health outcomes?

The high health outcomes solution pathways have low GINI (low income inequality) as a necessary condition. In the first pathway ~GINI is combined with higher levels of pre-secondary education only, along with very high consistency (0.867) and covers four countries. The second pathway (if consistency below 0.8 is allowed) combines ~GINI with higher levels of health expenditure, but also higher behavioural factors, and covers three countries, but with one deviant for consistency. Given its higher consistency and coverage, there are good grounds for seeing the first solution pathway as both empirically and substantively the most important.

What the necessary condition and subsequent sufficient solutions suggest is that in line with the work of Marmot and others, low income inequality is the most important social determinant factor in terms of achieving low health outcomes. Its combination with an education factor, which we would not assume would lead to high health outcomes, demonstrates the importance of conjunctional causation in that this factor, treated as an independent variable, is linked to poorer health outcomes in OECD research, but when combined with low GINI, for France, the Netherlands, Norway and Sweden, it does not.

In the context of those countries, it would seem that the disadvantage of lower levels of education is not sufficient to negate the advantage of low income inequality.

Germany, as noted earlier, is a deviant case for consistency in the high health outcomes solution. What this means is that Germany has a pattern of causal factors associated with high health outcomes, but falls instead into the low health outcomes achievement set (having a Commonwealth Fund score of −0.18). Deviant cases do not invalidate results because, although it is a reasonable assumption that the world has causes and effects which are more or less reliably present, our knowledge of the world will always be partial, and our measures of the world will always be less than perfect. QCA is a method designed to look for patterns in the data, but it is not possible to include every causal factor in models, and measurements are not 100 per cent reliable. However, deviant cases must be accounted for when they arise, and there is a clear case here for having to explore Germany in greater depth towards that goal.

Looking in more detail at Germany's health outcome measures shows that it scores particularly badly in relation to life expectancy at 60 years (second worse only to the US), and for its 30-day mortality rates after heart attacks (the worst of all the countries in the sample). There is the sense of a story emerging, when combined with Germany's poor behavioural factors, of older people dying earlier than in other countries because of circulatory problems. This is backed up the OECD health country profile, which notes Germany's lower than average life expectancy in Western Europe, and of the prevalence of heart disease there (OECD and Policies, 2019a). It also appears that heart disease mortality is actually rising. In contrast to the other two countries with which Germany shares the same pattern of social determinant factors on the truth table row, mortality from heart disease in the Netherlands is the second lowest in the EU (after France) (OECD and Policies, 2019b), and Switzerland has the second-highest life expectancy at 60 years. All three countries share poor results in terms of 30-day mortality rates after heart attacks, but the key factor of difference is that Germany does substantially worse in terms of mortality amenable to healthcare than either the Netherlands or Switzerland (83 per 100,000 for Germany, but 72 for the Netherlands and 55 for Switzerland). It would seem that although the behavioural factors (smoking and drinking) are similar across the three countries, Germany's health system is struggling to manage their implications, for older people especially, and in relation to preventable mortality for heart disease specifically.

As such, two main findings emerge in relation to existing work. First, the existence of low income inequality (~GINI) suggests it has a strong 'root' in the causation chains, leading to good health outcomes. Low GINI is able to work alongside both high tobacco and alcohol consumption and still generate high health outcomes in one solution pathway, and, in combination with low alcohol and high health expenditure, work alongside high numbers of low education attainment in another.

As well as Germany being deviant for consistency, there is one country which is deviant for coverage in the solution – Australia. What this means is that Australia has a set of social determinants which do not consistently have set-theoretical relationships with high health outcomes – but still achieves high health outcomes anyway.

Looking at the data at the beginning of the results section for health outcomes, ~GINI appears in all but one of the countries with high health outcomes. Of those countries, Australia, France, the Netherlands, Norway, Sweden and Switzerland, only one has high income inequality – Australia. Australia is therefore unusual in achieving high health outcomes given its pattern of social determinant factors, but especially in relation to achieving them with high income inequality.

Australia's success in terms of health outcomes is the most difficult case to account for in the sample here. It is a relatively low spender on healthcare, and has relatively high income inequality. In its favour it has low smoking rates, whereas its alcohol consumption levels are in the middle of the range of the countries here, so overall its behavioural factors are low.

Australia's success is credited by the World Health Organization as being due to its successes in public health – which are remarkable given its relatively low spend in this area (see Chapter 4). Australia is commended for its public health programmes (especially in relation to smoking reduction), campaigns to reduce coronary heart disease, its public health HIV response, and its strong health information infrastructure (Healy et al, 2006). These claims are borne out in the Commonwealth Fund health outcomes measures, where Australia scores strongly – but again subject to the differences between the predominantly white and indigenous populations.

However, considering Australia in its wider context gives us some more clues as to the relationships between its social determinants, which seem to be unpromising (except for behavioural factors) and its success in terms of health outcomes. A key part of this is that Australia's social determinants are significantly divergent between its white and its indigenous populations, with average gaps of around

10 per cent in income between the two groups across almost every age and every geography.[2] Twice as many indigenous Australians (45 per cent) receive income support compared to 23 per cent for the rest of the population. Nearly half of indigenous Australians report they could not raise $2000 in the event of an emergency compared to just over 10 per cent for non-indigenous groups. Nearly 40 per cent of the indigenous population are daily smokers, compared to just over 10 per cent for non-indigenous Australians.[3] There is a life expectancy gap of around eight years between the two groups[4] and significant gaps in terms of school attendance and achievement in all measures.[5]

What these factors point to is that Australia's social determinants are significantly divergent between different population groups. The indigenous population is around 3.3 per cent of the total, which is a relatively small proportion, but with such income and education inequalities, the 'gaps' between that group and the rest of Australians docs lead to an effect on its social determinant factors. In this context, Australia's health outcomes are remarkable – but if it were able to make more progress in terms of supporting the health of its indigenous people, it would achieve even more.

In terms of high health equity, one solution pathway appears to have the strongest empirical and theoretical support – that which combines a low GINI coefficient and high health expenditure, and which covers Norway, Sweden, Germany, Switzerland and the Netherlands. This solution term is an even stronger theoretical fit than the one for the same countries for health outcomes, as the education term (higher levels of pre-secondary education) is replaced with one that is a better fit with existing theory and research, higher health expenditures. This solution pathway is highly consistent (0.877) and has the highest unique coverage of those making up the overall solution.

Across these solutions, with the UK excepted, the combination of low GINI and high expenditure appears across the five cases. This finding combines insights from the social determinants literature (low GINI) with those from Deaton (2015) and OECD (2017) research in terms of the importance of health expenditure. It seems that, for the countries explored in this book, low income inequality and high health expenditure are sufficient for health equity.

There is one other pathway to high health equity, covering the UK only, and which has two factors we might have assumed would work against strong health equity – high behavioural factors, and high levels of income inequality. To understand why the UK achieves high health equity, it would seem we need to look for other causal factors. The

UK is not a deviant case, but its success in terms of health equity does require explanation.

Perhaps the simplest explanation of the UK's success with health equity, despite its social determinants measures of a combination of high behavioural factors and high income inequality, is the existence of its National Health Service (NHS). The NHS was characterised by Klein (1986) as a socialist health system which conservatives support (because of its high public support, the ability of governments to decentralise rationing and blame away from themselves to doctors), and this remains a powerful explanation. The NHS is a feature of British life, forming a central part of its 2012 Olympics opening ceremony, and during the COVID-19 pandemic a 'clap for carers' was instigated every Thursday at 8pm. Voluntary health insurance rates in the UK remain fairly low (making up 6 per cent of total health funding) and because of the principle of allocating care on the basis of need, it delivers care in a form which is largely the same, geographic differences excluded, for everyone. The NHS, then, achieves health equity, despite the UK's pattern of social determinants, because of its egalitarian approach to funding and access, with the vast majority of the population depending on it entirely for their healthcare.

In terms of both equity AND health outcomes, the combination of low income inequality and high levels of health spending are a necessary condition that is shared by all the countries in the solution set. As such ~GINI*CURREXP, because this combination is highly credible in terms of existing research, along with its statistical consistency and relevance, forms the core of solutions for countries achieving the combined outcome.

The sufficient solution appears to suggest that, although high levels of low education may result in poorer health outcomes, this negative effect is offset by the other three solution terms. The solution term here is highly consistent (0.876) and has a high unique coverage of the overall set (0.685), suggesting it has high credibility.

Switzerland, along with Norway, Sweden and the Netherlands, has both high health outcomes and high health equity but does not meet the consistency threshold from the solution term as its pattern of causal factors is shared by Germany, which scores in the low set for health outcomes. In common with Norway, Sweden and the Netherlands (as well as Germany), Switzerland has low income inequality and high health expenditure – the necessary factors for the combined outcome measure set. Switzerland differs in that, in the solution for high equity and high health outcomes, the Netherlands, Norway and Sweden have high levels of pre-secondary education only, whereas Switzerland has low levels – which is a better theoretical fit for both high health outcomes and high health equity. As such, although Switzerland is a deviant case in terms of the sufficient solution, its combination of social determinants factors is an even better theoretical fit for the achievement of the combined outcome. In contrast to Germany, with which it shares causal conditions, Switzerland achieves much better life expectancy at 60 years and has much better mortality amenable to healthcare. It seems, then, that Germany could learn from the Swiss healthcare system in its treatment of older people and the conditions they are more likely to experience as a result of their high behavioural factors – a topic already discussed earlier.

Conclusion

The social determinants of health represent a crucial first perspective on the effectiveness of health systems. This chapter has explored the social determinants of health in relation to several of the key factors which OECD research, and leading authors in the field, suggest are of the most importance in relation to health outcomes and health equity. The analysis could not include every possible social determinant but does give some clear findings about which factors appear to the most important when considered conjunctionally.

In terms of achieving either high health outcomes or high health equity, low income inequality (~GINI) was found to be a necessary condition, with ~GINI also appearing in both sufficient solutions for high health outcomes, and in the solution terms for five of the six countries (the UK excepted) for high health equity. There are therefore strong grounds for considering low income inequality as forming a crucial core around which conjunctional solutions can build. In Chapter 6, the most factors which appear to be most important in solution terms from each chapter will be brought together, and because of its importance here, income inequality will be the first of those factors.

For both high health outcomes and high health equity, ~GINI was also a necessary condition, but so was high health expenditure and so HEALTHEXP is also carried forward to Chapter 6, especially as existing research provides very strong evidence that high health expenditure is of such central importance in understanding the differences in life expectancy between different nations. The four countries which achieve both high health equity and high health outcomes are the Netherlands, Norway, Sweden and Switzerland, and although the necessary condition (~GINI*HEALTHEXP) covers all four nations, the sufficient solution covers three only, with Switzerland missing because of having the same combination of social determinant factors as Germany.

Germany is an important country in terms of the social determinants of health because it has a similar mix of factors as Switzerland, but it falls short of the achievement of Switzerland in terms of its health outcomes. Although both countries have behavioural factors which would suggest a more proactive public health strategy might be more appropriate, by digging deeper into the health outcomes measure Germany's lower than average life expectancy for older people and its prevalence of heart disease seem to be areas that policymakers need to especially address.

If Germany is perhaps doing worse in terms of health outcomes than we might expect, as it has the same mix of factors as Switzerland which is among the highest-performing countries, then Australia represents in many respects the opposite situation. Australia appears to succeed *despite* its social determinants – it has relatively high income inequality, high levels of pre-secondary education only, and is a relatively low spender on healthcare – its social determinants put it in the opposite set to Switzerland and Germany for every factor. This means that Australia does well on behavioural factors, but relatively poorly in all the others. In terms of social determinants alone, Australia's strong health outcomes are difficult to explain, but the sharply divergent results between its white and indigenous people is clearly a crucial factor that policymakers need to exert even greater energy in addressing.

In all then, this chapter has shown the power of the social determinants of health in addressing two key Commonwealth Fund outcome measures – for health outcomes and for health equity – and has highlighted the key role that two factors – income inequality and health expenditure – have in addressing them. The next chapter moves on to consider the role the different means of health funding play in achieving access to health services, and efficiency in their operation.

Before moving to the next chapter, three more detailed country case studies will be presented, those for Germany, Switzerland and Australia – three countries that came up as deviant in one form or another in the earlier analysis.

Case studies

Germany

The German health system is funded through mandatory health insurance, with nearly 90 per cent of the population enrolled in a scheme that covers hospital treatment (inpatient and outpatient), mental health and prescription drugs. Sickness funds administer the health system and are financed by general wage contributions shared by workers and employers. Despite the extensive public funding, co-payments are also made for inpatient services and drugs. Germans on higher incomes can opt out of the social health insurance system as long as they take out private health insurance instead. However, both sickness funds and private health insurers use the same healthcare providers, who treat all patients regardless of whether they are state funded or funded through private insurance, with the system as a whole being based on the principles of solidarity and subsidiarity. The state does not offer subsidies for private insurance and has almost no role in the delivery of healthcare.

The German healthcare system has shared decision making going across federal and state governments, as well as organisations representing payers and providers. As such, it is rather corporatist in structure, a system which makes for strong continuity, but which can sometimes make change difficult.

The German health system is well funded, with around three quarters of the financing coming from the public purse. There are a large number of sickness funds, many of which have links to particular occupations or groups, but with those links having become looser in recent years. The sickness funds are financed through compulsory wage contributions, with dependents being covered free of charge, and the wage contributions being pooled centrally into a health fund and reallocated to the individual sickness funds using a risk-based capitation formula. The sickness funds have also been encouraged to contract directly with providers in recent years (rather than using collective regional agreements) to attempt to increase competition and drive care efficiency. In addition to the compulsory wage contributions, there is also a much smaller income-dependent contribution to the costs of healthcare.

Private health insurance can be taken out by those on higher incomes and may be attractive for lower-risk groups (such as younger people on high incomes) who receive lifetime underwriting based on their risk at entry.

Out-of-pocket payments in Germany are common but not comparatively high, with spending typically going on medical goods, but with co-payments also in place (at a low rate) for hospital stays. Germany's health funding fuzzy-set scores are as follows:

COUNTRY	GOV	HEALTHEXP	OOP	VOL
GER	0.94	0.83	0.35	0.08

From this, Germany is a relatively high healthcare spender and is also a high spender in terms of government and compulsory insurance. On the other hand, it makes relatively little use of voluntary health insurance.

The public have a free choice of GPs and specialists, and there are no real gatekeepers to the system in place. Public and private hospitals have around half of beds each, with the private not-for-profit being larger than the for-profit sector, albeit with the latter undergoing growth.

Long-term care insurance is mandatory and provided by the same insurers that provide the social health insurance system, with employers and employees sharing the costs. This leads to a range of benefits being available for both home and institutional care through both cash payment and discounted long-term care services.

Germany's health expenditure fuzzy-set scores are as follows:

COUNTRY	HEALTHEXP	CUREREHAB	LONG	PREVENT
GER	0.83	0.28	0.35	0.57

From this, Germany is a relatively low spender on curative and rehabilitative services, as well as on long-term care. However, it falls into the high set of countries for preventative care.

Germany has the Robert Koch Institute, which reports to the Federal Ministry of Health, responsible for infectious diseases, as well as being heavily involved in epidemiological research and public health. Its role has been lauded in Germany's response to COVID, with the UK explicitly seeking to replicate it as a part of its public health strategy post COVID.

Germany's health system is one with a strong equity component with low unmet need, and its health insurance system is able to cover the needs of its population in a way that makes little difference between public and private holders of insurance.

Germany, then, has a highly equitable and well-funded and organised health service. However, in terms of the social determinants of health, the system faces some significant challenges in terms of behavioural factors, with higher levels of alcohol and tobacco consumption, but unlike the two countries which share its causal factors (Switzerland and France), it falls into the low health outcomes set. Germany has a relatively low health outcomes score, with life expectancy at age 60 at 23.7, a couple of years below Switzerland and France, while its mortality amenable to healthcare is higher than those two countries (83 per 100,000, with Switzerland at 55 and France 61), and its 30-day mortality rate after myocardial infarction is the worst of all the 11 countries in this book. This seems to point to older people, as well as those receiving treatment, not having as good health outcomes as those in other countries, and this may be related to the behavioural factor problems identified earlier and the challenge they present to the healthcare system not being fully met.

Germany's social determinants of health fuzzy-set scores are as follows:

COUNTRY	GINI	BEHAV	EDUC	HEALTHEXP
GER	0.13	0.93	0.23	0.83

Germany, then, is a relatively high spender on healthcare with low income inequalities and a low number of people with pre-secondary education only. However, its behavioural factors are very high because of its higher levels of smoking and drinking.

Switzerland

Switzerland has a highly decentralised health system, funded by its residents purchasing insurance from not-for-profit insurers, through taxes levied at the canton (effectively state) level, through social insurance contributions and through taxes at the municipal and federal levels. Public finance represents just under two thirds of all funding sources. Public coverage includes the majority of doctor visits, hospital care, medical goods (include pharmaceuticals), home care, long-term care, and physiotherapy. Individuals pay premiums to the insurer of their choice, but with funds being redistributed among insurers centrally, with a risk-equalisation scheme in place that adjusts for canton, age, gender and previous levels of expenditure. It is possible to gain a greater choice of physicians or access to improved hospital facilities by paying supplementary private insurance.

Under the mandatory health insurance scheme, insurers have a minimum annual deductible for adults, but can accept a higher level of deductible in return for a lower premium. In addition, people pay a 10 per cent fee for all services (coinsurance) subject to a cap of around $600 for adults and $300 for children. There are also charges for hospital stays (around $10 per night).

The federal and canton government offer income-based subsidies to help cover mandatory health insurance premiums, with around a quarter of people receiving them overall, but with substantial differences between cantons.

Citizens (including dependents) are legally required to purchase insurance, with cantons empowered to ensure compliance. The 26 cantons have their own constitutions and license providers, as well as coordinating hospital services and engaging in health promotion activities. They also subsidise premiums and institutions, where needed. Each canton has its own elected minister of public health.

The federal government regulates the finance for the overall system, as well as putting in place quality standards for medical goods, and assessments of the cost-effectiveness of the services being offered.

Switzerland's fuzzy-set scores for health funding are as follows:

COUNTRY	GOV	HEALTHEXP	OOP	VOL
SWI	0.03	1.00	1.00	0.59

The Swiss healthcare system is an extreme among the cases included in the book. It is a very high overall spender, with extremely low levels of government expenditure, and has high levels of voluntary health insurance and very high levels of out-of-pocket funding. This is a rather unusual combination of funding factors, but has some commonalities with the US.

The municipalities organise long-term care. The Swiss health expenditure fuzzy-set scores are as follows:

COUNTRY	HEALTHEXP	CUREREHAB	LONG	PREVENT
SWI	1.00	0.69	0.64	0.24

Switzerland is a comparatively very high spender on healthcare, as well as a high spender on curative and rehabilitative expenditure and on long-term care. It spends relatively less on preventative care however.

Switzerland's scores for social determinants are as follows:

COUNTRY	GINI	BEHAV	EDUC	HEALTHEXP
SWI	0.15	0.86	0.19	1.00

From these, Switzerland has relatively low income inequality, which is perhaps a surprise because of its reputation as being a financial centre, and also has low levels of people with pre-secondary education only. However, Switzerland has high levels of both smoking and drinking, and especially of smoking.

Australia

Australia has a complex and unusual health system. It has in place a regionally organised, universal public health insurance programme (called Medicare) that is financed through a combination of general taxation and government levy. All Australian citizens are automatically enrolled in Medicare and receive the right to free public hospital care, along with substantial coverage for doctor services and pharmaceutical expenditures. In addition, citizens from New Zealand (and other countries with reciprocal benefits) can also enrol in Medicare. However, half of Australians also purchase private supplementary insurance in order to be able to access the private hospital system, along with other services such as dentistry, with the federal government paying a rebate towards private insurance premiums, and also charging, on a means-tested basis, households that do not purchase private insurance.

Australia spends just over 10 per cent of GDP on healthcare, with two thirds of expenditures funded by the government, and Medicare being funded through the national tax system. Private health insurance is widely available and covers out-of-pocket fees and private providers, with the aim to achieve greater choice for patients (especially in relation to hospitals) and faster access for non-emergency care. There are caps for a range of services, and for hospital services patients can opt to be treated as public patients, where they receive full fee coverage, but probably longer waiting times, or private patients, where they receive 75 per cent fee coverage.

The federal government funds inpatient and outpatient care and pharmaceuticals, along with having a regulation role in relation to private health insurance. However, it plays very little role in direct service delivery.

Tax rebates for private health insurance make it attractive to people who can afford it, but there is an income-related penalty payment for those that choose not to hold it (which is means tested). There are also opportunities for younger people to commit to enrolling in private health insurance for life, but with a penalty on the premiums for each year after age 30.

Nearly 50 per cent of Australians have some kind of private health insurance, but with coverage varying by socio-economic status and skewed towards higher income groups, who are incentivised to join because of the imposition of a surcharge should they not do so.

Australia's fuzzy set scores for funding are as follows:

COUNTRY	GOVCOMP	HEALTHEXP	OOP	VOLPC
AUS	0.11	0.30	0.75	0.89

Australia is therefore a comparatively low spender overall and has a relatively low level of government funding for its health system.

However, it has high levels of out-of-pocket payments and voluntary health insurance.

State governments both own and manage the delivery of public hospitals, along with ambulances, dental care, community care (predominately primary care and preventative care) and providing mental health services. State governments are funded through their own finance systems, as well as receiving federal funding. State governments also regulate private hospitals and engage in health planning in relation to the location of pharmacies and the health workforce.

State governments are also involved in the delivery of community health and preventative health programmes. Australia's health expenditure fuzzy-set scores are as follows:

COUNTRY	HEALTHEXP	CUREREHAB	LONG	PREVENT
AUS	0.30	0.98	0.02	0.03

Australia has very high curative and rehabilitative expenditure, but spends relatively very little on long-term care or preventative care. Its mix of expenditure is unlike any other country in this sample.

Australia, then, is a complex mix. On the one hand it can claim to be, because of Medicare, a universal, public health system. But there are strong incentives, especially for the better off, to also take out private health insurance, which is likely to result in quicker treatment and access to better-funded private hospitals. This results in a fairly visible two-tier system, with socio-economic status dividing the groups.

The greatest gaps in health outcomes are between the Aboriginal and Torres Strait Islander groups, and the rest of the Australian population. Life expectancy gaps are around 10 years between those communities, with government targets to narrow the gaps struggling to make progress.

In the account just presented, we can begin to get an idea of the reasons for Australia's very distinctive mix of causal factors. Australia's very liberal economy is linked to its relatively high income inequality, and its difficulty in fully confronting its past around its Aboriginal and Torres Strait Islander groups helps explain its relatively poor performance in relation to both education and alcohol consumption – but with the latter also having strong roots in its links to recreational situations for other groups as well. Although Australia has its Medicare system, its government expenditure levels are comparatively low, and its out-of-pocket and voluntary health insurance levels relatively high, underpinned by extensive means testing but concerns about a two-tier system between public and private. The mix of public and private systems is dealt with far more efficiently than in the US in terms of administration, but is less efficient than highly public systems such as those of the UK and Norway. Australia has the lowest long-term expenditures of any country in the sample here and is underpinned by a complex mixed economy of informal and formal care being paid for by a mix of public (means-tested) and private finance.

In terms of health outcomes, Australia's mix of public (means-tested) care and incentivised private insurance appears to work well. However, in terms of health equity, and despite significant efforts to close health gaps between the Aboriginal and Torres Strait Islanders and the rest of the population, it is clearly facing significant challenges and progress is stalling. However, Australia does appear to offer lessons to other countries with significant public-private mixes in place, especially the US, which does poorly across most of the measures in which Australia scores highly. Australia appears to demonstrate that healthcare costs can be contained (despite significant concerns about financing within the country) and that systems of means testing can be put in place that still achieve high health outcomes.

In terms of social determinants, Australia's fuzzy-set scores are as follows:

COUNTRY	GINI	BEHAV	EDUC	HEALTHEXP
AUS	0.68	0.28	0.85	0.30

Australia has relatively high income inequality and also a high number of people with pre-secondary education only. However, it does have relatively low behavioural factors. The overall behavioural score slightly conceals the actual situation though, with among the lowest levels of smoking in the sample, but relatively high alcohol consumption.

3

Healthcare funding

Introduction

The way in which health systems are funded is often based on a series of political decisions which were made in the early development of different nations' health systems, and yet, through processes of institutional reproduction, have remained remarkably intact today (Immergut, 1992b; Wilsford, 1995). As health systems absorb such substantial levels of resources, and because access to healthcare is not only recognised as a human right, but is also an international business of enormous scale, methods of healthcare funding in a particular country will be the result of a series of compromises between competing interests. Key stakeholders are those working in health services (with doctors usually having the most influence), government, public, private or not-for-profit providers of care, as well as other organisations such as insurance companies, patient representative groups and regulatory bodies. At election time the public will also have a say, but generally only from the 'menu' of options presented to them. Should events occur with particular salience to the general public (such as a rogue doctor or nurse, or a vulnerable person not receiving the right care), this can also mobilise change, especially should those events occur near an election.

This chapter explores the different configurations of the funding of health systems among the 11 countries included in the book, and the relationship between these configurations and access to healthcare, as well as a measure of the efficiency of the health system.

It therefore aims to discover whether there are patterns of healthcare funding that have necessary or sufficient relationships with healthcare access and measured efficiency, as well as whether there are any health systems which achieve both of these outcomes.

Healthcare funding

Healthcare is funded through a range of sources, but at the highest level of abstraction this involves a mix of money from the government, from health insurance of various kinds, or from the public through private, out-of-pocket payments. Government-funded health systems may utilise compulsory social health insurance as well as general taxation as their source of money. Health insurance can be public (where it can turn into a government scheme), or be organised on a private or not-for-profit basis. Out-of-pocket payments can be used to supplement government funding or insurance-based systems. Health funding involves a complex mix of different sources, all of which are present in some form in almost every health system.

All the health systems explored in this chapter have significant government funding, with healthcare being acknowledged to carry with it a range of justifications for public funding. Access to healthcare is regarded by the World Health Organization as a universal right, with that right being framed in its 1946 Constitution, but different countries have different levels of commitment to access, and very different ways of achieving it. Governments do not wish to see their injured or ill citizens being unable to receive care and treatment, and this means some state-based funding will always be needed, unless an alternative to public funding can be found based entirely on charitable donations. There are also clear collective incentives to publicly fund programmes based around vaccinations to achieve as high a take-up as possible. At the same time, government funding may be a pragmatic recognition that poor health can simply be the result of bad luck, creating a reason to 'pool risk', funding healthcare through either general taxation or compulsory insurance payments in which everyone pays in, but from which everyone can also draw should they need care.

Funding healthcare publicly means that the government is able to set an overall budget and achieve a degree of accountability and control over it. This has advantages in that it might lead to efficiencies through the avoidance of complex insurance billing arrangements, as well as giving the opportunity for a single body to have oversight over health funding.

However, funding health services through the public purse can also mean that the growth of health services is slower than it might be through other means, as health is only one government department competing for taxation revenues, with the risk of demand for healthcare outstripping supply, and of waiting lists for treatments increasing as a result. There is also the risk of public organisation leading to the creation of large bureaucracies which may be less efficient and less responsive to public need than would ideally be the case.

Opponents of public funding for healthcare point to other potential disadvantages. If healthcare is funded through general taxation and everyone is given access to it as a result, then there is a risk of 'moral hazard', of people overusing the service, or even not looking after their health as well as they might have done if they had paid for healthcare access themselves. These arguments point to the need for there to be a link between personal responsibility and the way healthcare is funded, and to suggestions that this needs to be taken into greater consideration.

Insurance schemes can be compulsory or voluntary, and public, private or not-for-profit, or a mix of them all. This makes health insurance difficult to categorise and theorise about. Health insurance, at the abstract level, means that in return for a payment, which is either rated at the individual or community level, an individual receives the ability to access a defined amount of healthcare in return should they need it. However, beyond that abstraction lies the questions of who pays the premium, and at what rate. The premium can be paid by individual people, the government, or their employer (if they have one), or a mix of all three. If insurance is rated at the community level, people will pay a premium based on the average need of people in that community. If the premium is rated at the individual level, it will be based on their own assessed health risk. Community rating attempts to deal with the possibility of bad luck, but may also carry a degree of moral hazard with it, in that it loosens the link between individual health behaviours and the premiums. Individual health premiums may emphasise personal responsibility more strongly, but high-risk groups may not be able to afford to pay them, potentially leaving people underinsured or uninsured for the care they might need.

If health insurance is compulsory it operates in a similar way to government funding, and indeed the OECD categorises the two in the same way in its own statistics. Social health insurance is often funded through compulsory work-based contributions, with groups out of work having access to government-subsidised compulsory insurance or a separate government scheme. However, in such systems, the funds are usually combined centrally in a similar way to taxation.

If health insurance is entirely private and voluntary, it is categorised in OECD health statistics separately from government and compulsory insurance, and typically operates through employers offering health insurance as an additional benefit (through which they may be able to access healthcare more quickly), or by individuals or families taking out their own health insurance plans on a non-compulsory basis. Such systems are still likely to have government funding for those that cannot afford to pay from their own resources, but there may still end up being gaps in provision for those that fail to meet the means test for government funding, but who cannot afford, or who choose not to have, private health insurance.

Finally, healthcare can be funded through out-of-pocket expenditures. As the name suggests, healthcare can often be purchased through private funds if people can afford to pay for it themselves. Out-of-pocket payments can cover the whole costs of care and often occur when people wish to have either quicker access or better healthcare facilities than might be available through state-funded systems. More often, however, co-payments occur alongside both public or insurance-based health systems so that people have to pay a share or at least a contribution towards the costs of healthcare. No health system in the book even comes close to having co-payments as the largest element of financing, with Switzerland having by far the largest out-of-pocket contributions per capita (see Chapter 1, Table 1.2). However, most health systems retain some aspect of out-of-pocket expenditures, considering it as a means of preventing overuse (by asking people to use their own funds, the assumption is that people will only use healthcare if they need to), or as a reflection that some people may simply be prepared, or be able, to pay more for healthcare than others. People may be prepared to use their own finances to buy access to quicker treatment, or be asked (though a means-tested system especially) to make a contribution to the costs of their healthcare by paying some of the cost of drugs or other treatments. However, extensive use of out-of-pocket payments may make healthcare unaffordable for people with few resources, and may also increase bureaucracy because it will tend to result in complex billing arrangements through its combination with means testing or other eligibility checking.

Issues and tensions in health funding

Health systems are also not independent of the wider governments and societies in which they function. This does not mean that health systems have to reflect the wider government, or the preferences of society, and the relationship between these elements will be complex, and linked to layered historical contingencies and power relationships. As noted earlier, institutions are created as the result of compromise decisions made by actors in a particular period of time, along with the often smaller changes governments have made since then. Changes are often layered onto old mechanisms, and existing mechanisms repurposed and converted to new ends. The health funding system in the US, with its dizzying complexity, is the result of the layering of changes, especially since the 1960s, and the complexity of which has become a barrier to attempts to change it because of the sheer difficulty in describing what such change would entail (Gordon, 2009).

Existing funding systems give resources and power to interests such as insurance companies, trade unions, medical representation groups and patient groups, all of whom who will lobby hard to prevent changes that might disadvantage them. Health systems often reflect the values of those who were able to create their institutions, albeit in highly compromised form, and may be difficult to change. Even when a consensus exists in society that health funding changes need to be made, it may be difficult to achieve sufficient agreement on what kind of change is needed, especially in the face of existing interests favoured by the present system lobbying hard. This is most visible in the failed attempt by President Clinton to change the US healthcare system in the 1990s, where it seems at the beginning of the process there was a societal consensus that significant change was needed, but in the face of intensive lobbying and the fracturing of agreement about the exact type of change, political divisions reopened and barriers were erected to prevent change (Skocpol, 1997). The subsequent passing of the ACA under President Obama can be seen as a conspicuous learning of the lessons of the Clinton era by engaging early with key political and medical interest groups, but also being fortunate in the legislative process due to an historical voting contingency in Congress (Starr, 2013). However, at the time of writing, the future of the ACA still remains in doubt.

There are different perspectives on health funding which frame the optimal balance between the three major sources of funding as well as linking those sources to access and efficiency in different ways.

The issue of access to health services, as noted earlier, raises complex questions around moral hazard that are also linked to service efficiency. Moral hazard occurs where an individual is protected in some way from the consequences of their actions, and so is insulated from the risks that their decision might entail. Moral hazard may occur in health systems that are funded primarily from public sources with low out-of-pocket payments, as people do not have to directly pay the costs of illness and so may over-consume healthcare by visiting health facilities when they do not need to, or by making appointments that they do not keep. All of these elements would detract from the efficiency of the health system. Moral hazard occurs also occurs with voluntary health insurance where people can take a view that, if they are going to pay for health insurance, then they will make sure they receive some benefit from it. Insurers try to guard against this by offering discounts for those who do not claim against their insurance, by having co-payments for healthcare, or in the context of healthcare specifically by offering discounts for those who are able to show they are maintaining high standards of health. Guarding against moral hazard, however, adds to the complexity of the bureaucracy administering the system, and so potentially has adverse effects on efficiency.

The institutional answer to moral hazard, then, is the use of out-of-pocket expenditures. These ask people to contribute to the costs of healthcare from their own private funds, so, the argument goes, making them calculate the costs and benefits of seeking treatment in line with their willingness to pay for it. This may help increase allocative efficiency but at the price of some people who cannot afford treatment not receiving it, or some ill people not being able to afford to pay for healthcare that might be beneficial for them. As such, the use of out-of-pocket payments might increase efficiency but risks reducing access by asking some people to pay who may be unable or unwilling to do so.

From the perspective of public choice theorists, there is a critique of the public sector which argues that, insulated from market pressures, public services are intrinsically less efficient than their private counterparts. If this argument is correct then health systems with a stronger private orientation should generate better efficiency, but also potentially better access as supply might more closely match demand.

However, claims of the public choice school do fly in the face of at least some existing evidence, with the US system being heavily privatised but scoring poorly for both efficiency and access, and with the predominantly publicly funded UK NHS achieving high scores in each category. Indeed, Conservative Chancellor Nigel Lawson came to regard the NHS as being extremely efficient because of its public funding, not despite it (Lawson, 1991).

Debates around health financing, then, are about the balance between the three different sources of health funding. Advocates of government-funded systems tend to present a theory that they should improve access and make healthcare provision more equitable. Those that argue for voluntary health insurance suggest that doing so will make healthcare more efficient as people will only take health coverage that they require, reducing costs and more closely matching need with health financing. In some countries (such as the UK), the use of out-of-pocket payments is politically controversial as it is regarded as preventing the poorest from accessing health services, even with means testing in place. This has resulted in a divergence in, for example, the use of charges for prescription medicine between England (which has a means-tested fee) and Scotland (in which prescriptions are free for everyone). However, anyone experiencing the Australian health system would be used to the idea of out-of-pocket fees being widely used and applying for exemptions or claiming proportions of fees paid back as a matter of routine.

The next section outlines the data used in the chapter.

The data for this chapter come from the OECD, which has a robust database of health funding statistics for all the countries in the book. The top level of categorisation for the OECD's health funding statistics divides funding sources into the three main categories discussed in the earlier review.

First, there are government and compulsory contributory healthcare financing schemes. These form the largest component of the different kinds of health funding here, but still vary in size from just under 50 per cent (the US) through to over 85 per cent (Norway). This category brings together schemes funded by general taxation, and/or those that instead use compulsory payroll taxes which pay into social insurance schemes.

The second main category is voluntary health insurance schemes, which is primarily made up of employer-based insurance (which is non-compulsory), government-based voluntary insurance, and community-based insurance. The key element of voluntary health insurance is that these schemes involve some degree of inter-personal or inter-temporal pooling, separating the time of payment and the time of service use.

Third, there are household out-of-pocket payments, both those that are based on cost sharing, and those that are not. Out-of-pocket expenditures involve, in OECD terminology, direct payment for healthcare goods from the household primary income or savings. These payments avoid the use of third parties and are typically made at the time of purchase of the goods or use of the service.

Although it is possible to disaggregate these headings further, they give us a strong basis to work from in exploring different health funding. For each of the funding sources the proportion of total health funding is used for government and compulsory insurance, and for voluntary health insurance, as both of these tend not to be directly paid for by individual people – they are funded either through taxation or through employment-based schemes. Using the proportional figures for these two sources gives us an idea of the relative size of these two sources of funding in relation to one another. For out-of-pocket expenditures, however, as they are paid for through household funds or saving, the per capita expenditures (US$ PPP) give a sense of the scale of personal expenditures required. It is also worth mentioning that analysis considering all the funding categories proportionally, and with total funding included as a proportion of GDP instead, produces very similar patterning of countries in terms of their 'fuzzy' attributes (Greener, 2020) and so leads to similar results.

In common with the other chapters of the book, the overall level of funding for health systems needs to be taken into account, and the spend per capita (US$ PPP), for each country is used.

The US represents a particular challenge in terms of its health funding categorisation. The US has seen the most significant change to its mode of health financing since the 1960s, when Medicare and Medicaid were established. The ACA led to a requirement for the public to hold health insurance through a complex scheme which has been implemented in an uneven way because of the refusal of many states to fully cooperate with it, because of a series of legal challenges to it, and because of the repeated attempts to undermine it during the presidency of Donald Trump.

The main issue is how we categorise the funding of the US system. The OECD measures for the US have been significantly changed since 2017 to account for the changes to the system, with some of the measures being recalculated from 2014 (at the time of writing) to try and show the new situation. That means that, again at the time of writing, the government and compulsory share of health financing moves from around 49 per cent in 2013 to 84 per cent in 2014, and voluntary health insurance moves from 39 per cent to just over 4 per cent over the same period. This clearly generates a substantial discontinuity in the data. At the same time, there is a definitional problem as to whether the ACA changes represent the introduction of compulsory health insurance or not, as much of the compulsion was removed during the long process of it becoming law and through subsequent legal challenges.

Given that the effects of the ACA on the US healthcare system will not appear for some time, and the lack of clarity over whether it represents the introduction of compulsory health insurance or not, the pre-ACA funding measures were used here, taken from a dataset produced by the OECD in 2017 which had not been updated to incorporate the new calculations. As such, the healthcare financing measures for the US categorise it in terms of being very low for government expenditure, high in terms of overall expenditure, high in terms of voluntary health insurance, and high in terms of out-of-pocket payments. However, in Chapter 6 a comparison with the post-ACA pattern of causal factors will be performed.

The calibrated fuzzy-set funding data for the 11 countries is shown in Table 3.1.

Table 3.1: Calibrated fuzzy-set data for health funding in 11 countries

COUNTRY	GOV	HEALTHEXP	OOP	VOL
Australia	0.11	0.30	0.75	0.83
Canada	0.20	0.33	0.36	0.95
France	0.76	0.24	0.02	0.93
Germany	0.94	0.83	0.35	0.07
Netherlands	0.85	0.76	0.31	0.24
New Zealand	0.82	0.02	0.06	0.26
Norway	0.95	0.99	0.84	0.03
Sweden	0.93	0.81	0.66	0.03
Switzerland	0.03	1.00	1.00	0.33
UK	0.77	0.08	0.25	0.19
US	0.00	1.00	0.97	1.00

From Table 3.1, the US generates a funding pattern at the extreme edges for every category, being extremely low in terms of government funding, but extremely high for overall health expenditure, out-of-pocket payments and voluntary health insurance. This health system is a high-spend, private one. If the US is a high-spend private system, Australia is a low-spend variation, with low government spending, low overall spend, but high out-of-pocket and high voluntary health insurance.

In many respects, New Zealand and the UK are the opposite of the US, with high government expenditure, but low overall levels of expenditure, out-of-pocket payments and voluntary health insurance. As such, New Zealand and the UK represent highly public health systems. Germany and the Netherlands are a high-spend variation of a public system, with high government funding and high health expenditure, but low out-of-pocket expenditure and voluntary health insurance. They have exactly the opposite pattern of funding to Australia.

Norway and Sweden are hybrids, with high government funding, high health expenditure, and out-of-pocket funding, but low voluntary health insurance. They therefore make relatively high use of both government and one private funding source – out-of-pocket expenditure – but low use of another private source – voluntary health insurance.

The way that countries 'cluster' in line with their fuzzy-set scores appears in Table 3.2.

Table 3.2: Fuzzy-set health funding clustering for 11 countries

GOV	HEALTHEXP	OOP	VOL	CASES
0	0	0	1	CAN
0	0	1	1	AUS
0	1	1	0	SWI
0	1	1	1	US
1	0	0	0	NZ, UK
1	0	0	1	FRA
1	1	0	0	GER, NLD
1	1	1	0	NOR, SWE

Each country's funding pattern here is in accordance with the combination of factors, which, when calculated in line with fuzzy logic, would achieve a score of over 0.5. For Canada, this combination would be ~GOV*~HEALTHEXP*~OOP*VOL, which from the calibrated data presented in Table 3.1 would be the minimum (*, in fuzzy logic requires us to take the minimum score in line with the logical AND) of 0.8, 0.67, 0.64 and 0.95, which is 0.64. That is the only combination of factors which would lead to a score of above 0.5 for Canada, and so is the combination which is shown in Table 3.2. This clustering of countries, following the previous paragraph, groups New Zealand and the UK as having the same causal combination, as do (with different combinations) Germany and the Netherlands, and Norway and Sweden.

In terms of directional expectations, for high access high government spending, low voluntary health insurance and low out-of-pocket expenditures are all supported by existing research and theory. High government expenditure should lead to wider access for groups that cannot afford to pay market rates for care, and lower levels of both voluntary health insurance and out-of-pocket payments should mean that relatively poorer groups do not have to pay for care from their own resources.

For high efficiency, in line with existing claims by policymakers such as Lawson (1991), directional expectations of high government spending and low voluntary health insurance were incorporated. High government spending should lead to greater efficiency where economies of scale and central cost control can be applied, and low voluntary health insurance should reduce the need to employ teams of people to assess and make decisions on insurance payments, as well as reduce the time of medical professionals in having to deal with such bureaucracy. However, as noted in Chapter 2, these directional expectations only affect the intermediate solution, and do not exclude empirically observed data from the calculations of sufficient solutions, being concerned with counterfactual rows of the truth table only.

High health access

The calibrated data for the 11 countries in relation to the scores for access to healthcare are shown in Table 3.3.

Table 3.3 shows that the high access countries are Australia, Germany, the Netherlands, New Zealand (which is just over the 0.5 threshold), Norway, Sweden and the UK, with the highest scores for the Netherlands and Germany. The lowest access scores go to Canada and the US.

In the analysis of necessary conditions, the two nearest candidates were GOV (high government funding), which has a consistency of 0.8 and a relevance of 0.76, and ~VOL (low levels of voluntary insurance), which has a consistency of 0.81 and a relevance of 0.8. GOV is a clear fit with existing research for achieving better access, and so was included in the calculation of the sufficient results in this chapter. Equally, ~VOL fits with existing theory as high voluntary insurance could prevent low-income groups from accessing some health services.

Table 3.3: High access and health funding fuzzy-set scores

COUNTRY	GOV	HEALTHEXP	OOP	VOL	ACCESS
Australia	0.11	0.30	0.75	0.83	0.72
Canada	0.20	0.33	0.36	0.95	0.04
France	0.76	0.24	0.02	0.93	0.36
Germany	0.94	0.83	0.35	0.07	0.95
Netherlands	0.85	0.76	0.31	0.25	0.97
New Zealand	0.82	0.02	0.06	0.26	0.52
Norway	0.95	0.99	0.84	0.03	0.67
Sweden	0.93	0.81	0.66	0.03	0.57
Switzerland	0.03	1.00	1.00	0.33	0.39
UK	0.77	0.08	0.25	0.19	0.87
US	0.00	1.00	0.97	1.00	0.01

Table 3.4: Truth table for high health access and health funding

GOV	CURREXP	OOP	VOL	OUT	Consistency	PRI	Cases
0	0	0	1	0	0.654	0.230	CAN
0	0	1	1	0	0.798	0.652	AUS
0	1	1	0	0	0.778	0.292	SWI
0	1	1	1	0	0.461	0.099	US
1	0	0	0	1	0.904	0.817	NZ, UK
1	0	0	1	0	0.699	0.336	FRA
1	1	0	0	1	0.996	0.993	GER, NLD
1	1	1	0	1	0.891	0.797	NOR, SWE

Looking across the high-access countries, Germany, the Netherlands, New Zealand, Norway and Sweden all have GOV*~VOL in common. However, one country – Australia – has high access but exactly the opposite combination ~GOV*VOL. This creates something of a dilemma – and two possible sufficient solutions for high access, one of which excludes Australia on the grounds that, as in the social determinants chapter, it appears as an outlier, and one which includes it. The differences this makes to the solution terms will be explained further later.

The full truth table, set with a consistency of 0.8 (but with the same truth table being produced up to 0.89) is set out in Table 3.4.

Table 3.4 builds on the data presented in the data section but including consistency scores. What it again emphasises is the dilemma that Australia offers – using a consistency threshold of 0.8, Australia is excluded from the sufficient solution. However, Australia's consistency score, despite having none of the necessary conditions, is 0.797 – a tiny amount beneath that 0.8 benchmark. The same truth table as Table 3.4 is produced with a consistency of up to 0.89 (with Norway and Sweden scoring 0.891). Australia's PRI score is 0.652, which would make it a strong candidate for inclusion and differentiates it from Switzerland, which has a consistency of 0.778, so only just below Australia, but has a PRI score of only 0.292, so falling below the 0.55/0.6 benchmark, which is a useful rule of thumb.

Given Australia's 'borderline' status, solutions which exclude and include Australia are presented, along with a comparison of the two.

First, if a consistency between 0.798 and 0.89 is used (so excluding Australia), with directional expectations of high government spending, and low out-of-pocket and low voluntary health insurance spending, then the following sufficient solution appears:

Solution	Consistency	PRI	Coverage	Unique coverage	Cases
GOV*HEALTHEXP*~VOL	0.857	0.789	0.525	0.170	GER, NLD, NOR, SWE
GOV*~OOP*~VOL	0.937	0.896	0.549	0.195	GER, NLD, NZ,UK
Solution consistency 0.854, Coverage 0.719					

The sufficient solution here offers two routes to high health access, but with considerable overlap between the two.

The first pathway combines high government spending with high health spending and low voluntary health insurance, and covers Germany, the Netherlands, Norway and Sweden.

The second pathway combines high government spending with low out-of-pocket spending and low voluntary health insurance, and covers Germany and the Netherlands (as with the first pathway), but also New Zealand and the UK. Both solution pathways have high consistency (with no deviant cases for consistency), and both contain the necessary condition identified of GOV*~VOL.

However, the solution is missing one of the countries with high access – so Australia is deviant for coverage. The conservative solution is the same as the previous one, with the parsimonious solution being simple GOV*~VOL, and so stressing again the necessary condition already identified.

If the consistency threshold is reduced to 0.797, then the intermediate solution changes to include Australia in a third solution pathway:

Solution	Consistency	PRI	Coverage	Unique coverage	Cases
GOV*HEALTHEXP*~VOL	0.857	0.789	0.525	0.170	GER, NLD, NOR, SWE
GOV*~OOP*~VOL	0.937	0.896	0.549	0.195	GER, NLD, NZ,UK
~GOV*~HEALTHEXP *OOP*VOL	0.798	0.652	0.209	0.099	AUS
Solution consistency 0.824, Coverage 0.818					

The conservative solution and parsimonious solution are identical to the intermediate solution here.

Comparing the two solutions, the first has a higher consistency (0.854 compared to 0.824), but lower coverage (0.719 compared to 0.818). However, the second solution includes a case (Australia) which has entirely the opposite set of funding factors that the analysis of necessary conditions suggested. These are the trade-offs for including Australia, which, as we saw in Chapter 2, was also the exception in the calculation of necessary conditions for high health outcomes and a case deviant for coverage in the high health outcomes solution there as well.

Results: high efficiency

The calibrated data for health funding and high efficiency are shown in Table 3.5.

The high efficiency countries are therefore Australia, Canada, Germany, New Zealand, Norway, Sweden and the UK, with France, the Netherlands, Switzerland and the US falling into the low efficiency set.

In calculating necessary conditions for high health efficiency, two combinations had both high consistency and relevance. GOV+~HEALTHEXP (high government funding and low overall levels of health expenditure with consistency 0.9, relevance 0.63), and GOV+~OOP (high government funding and low out-of-pockets funding with consistency 0.8, coverage 0.64) both produced statistically

Table 3.5: Calibrated dataset for high efficiency and health funding

COUNTRY	GOV	HEALTHEXP	OOP	VOL	EFFICIENCY
Australia	0.11	0.30	0.75	0.83	0.97
Canada	0.20	0.33	0.36	0.95	0.60
France	0.76	0.24	0.02	0.93	0.01
Germany	0.94	0.83	0.35	0.07	0.60
Netherlands	0.85	0.76	0.31	0.24	0.35
New Zealand	0.82	0.02	0.06	0.26	0.95
Norway	0.95	0.99	0.84	0.03	0.93
Sweden	0.93	0.81	0.66	0.03	0.78
Switzerland	0.03	1.00	1.00	0.33	0.38
UK	0.77	0.08	0.25	0.19	0.95
US	0.00	1.00	0.97	1.00	0.01

strong results which also make theoretical sense. High government spending might result in an efficient health system if economies of scale or scope could be achieved. Low overall health spending can also suggest an efficient system, if that system were spending less because it was efficient. Low out-of-pocket expenditure would also show potential efficiency as it might indicate the avoidance of potential duplication and bureaucracy that might occur in an out-of-pocket funding system.

Because the necessary conditions here contain the logical OR (+) they are a bit more complex.

In terms of the first necessary condition, GOV+~HEALTHEXP, Australia and Canada achieve this through ~HEALTHEXP only, Germany, Norway and Sweden achieve it through GOV only, and New Zealand and the UK achieve it through having both factors.

In terms of the second necessary condition, GOV+~OOP, Norway and Sweden achieve this through GOV only, and Canada through ~OOP only. Germany, New Zealand and the UK have both GOV and ~OOP. Once again, Australia appears to be the exception, having the combination of ~GOV+OOP – the opposite of the conditions outlined. This Australian exceptionalism matters less here as it matches the first necessary condition by having low health expenditure.

The truth table (Table 3.6) was generated with a consistency of 0.8, but produces the same solution up to 0.835.

Table 3.6 shows that there is another 'near-miss' row using a consistency threshold of 0.8, with Germany and the Nethrlands having a consistency of 0.788. The PRI score on that row is 0.534. From the calibrated data in Table 3.5, Germany does achieve high efficiency, but the Netherlands does not, and that suggests that there is something which separates those two countries which the truth table is not taking into account (or that Germany's score of 0.08 in the 'raw' Commonwealth Fund data makes it a marginal case as it achieves a result of just above zero). As Germany is such a marginal case, with its PRI score not meeting the 0.6 guideline used in examples by Dusa (2018), the sufficient results were calculated with the higher consistency threshold, and with directional expectations of high government spending and low voluntary health insurance, but with very similar solutions being generated with most directional combinations including high government spending.

The intermediate sufficient solution was as follows:

Table 3.6: Truth table for high health efficiency and health funding

GOV	HEALTHEXP	OOP	VOL	OUT	Consistency	PRI	Cases
0	0	0	1	1	0.836	0.702	CAN
0	0	1	1	1	0.987	0.976	AUS
0	1	1	0	0	0.762	0.358	SWI
0	1	1	1	0	0.574	0.236	US
1	0	0	0	1	0.971	0.956	NZ, UK
1	0	0	1	0	0.596	0.361	FRA
1	1	0	0	0	0.788	0.534	GER, NLD
1	1	1	0	1	0.992	0.985	NOR, SWE

Solution	Consistency	PRI	Coverage	Unique coverage	Cases
GOV*·HEALTHEXP*VOL	0.857	0.780	0.294	0.176	AUS, CAN
GOV*~HEALTHEXP *~OOP*~VOL	0.971	0.956	0.347	0.173	NZ, UK
GOV*HEALTHEXP *OOP*~VOL	0.992	0.985	0.377	0.244	NOR, SWE
Solution consistency 0.940, Coverage 0.767					

There are three solution pathways for high efficiency.

The first pathway combines low government expenditure with low health expenditure and low voluntary health insurance, and covers the cases of Australia and Canada.

The second pathway combines high government spending with low health expenditure, low out-of-pocket expenditure and low voluntary health insurance, and covers the cases of New Zealand and the UK.

The third solution pathway combines high government expenditure with high health expenditure, high out-of-pocket expenditure and low voluntary health insurance. It covers the cases of Norway and Sweden.

The conservative solution is identical, whereas the parsimonious solution still has three pathways, but simplifies the solution term for Norway and Sweden (pathway 3) to GOV*OOP, the pathway for Australia and Canada to ~GOV*~HEALTHEXP*VOL, and the pathway for New Zealand and the UK to GOV*~HEALTHEXP*VOL.

From the analysis of the truth table, Germany is a case deviant for coverage, and so is measured as having high efficiency, but does not appear in the solution, but there are no cases deviant for consistency.

If the truth table consistency is reduced to 0.787, the following intermediate solution appears:

Solution	Consistency	PRI	Coverage	Unique coverage	Cases
GOV*HEALTHEXP*~VOL	0.795	0.696	0.453	0.192	GER, NLD, NOR, SWE
GOV*~OOP*~VOL	0.871	0.805	0.475	0.173	GER, NLD, NZ, UK
~GOV*~HEALTHEXP*VOL	0.857	0.780	0.294	0.176	AUS, CAN
Solution consistency 0.844, Coverage 0.843					

The first pathway here presents Germany, the Netherlands, Norway and Sweden as clustered around high government funding, high health expenditure and low voluntary health insurance. It is similar to the third pathway of the first solution but removes high out-of-pocket funding to increase the coverage to include Germany and the Netherlands. However, the Netherlands is a case deviant for consistency.

The second solution pathway combines Germany and the Netherlands with New Zealand and the UK through the combination of high government funding, low out-of-pocket funding and low voluntary health insurance. It is similar to the second pathway in the first solution which also covers New Zealand and the UK, but removes low health expenditure to expand its coverage to include Germany and the Netherlands. However, the Netherlands is again deviant for consistency.

The third pathway is for Australia and Canada, and has the same configuration as in the first solution.

The two QCA solutions therefore give a choice – of either accounting for Germany as a case deviant for coverage (as in the first of the two solutions), or the Netherlands as a case deviant for consistency (as in the second solution), with the former solution being more consistent, but the latter having greater coverage.

The next section explores countries achieving both high access and high efficiency – which may offer a means of exploring which of the solution pathways for efficiency survives the harder test of having to achieve both outcomes.

Table 3.7: Calibrated data for high access and efficiency, and health funding

COUNTRY	GOV	HEALTHEXP	OOP	VOL	ACCESS AND EFFICIENCY
Australia	0.11	0.30	0.75	0.83	0.72
Canada	0.20	0.33	0.36	0.95	0.04
France	0.76	0.24	0.02	0.93	0.01
Germany	0.94	0.83	0.35	0.07	0.60
Netherlands	0.85	0.76	0.31	0.25	0.35
New Zealand	0.82	0.02	0.06	0.26	0.52
Norway	0.95	0.99	0.84	0.03	0.67
Sweden	0.93	0.81	0.66	0.03	0.57
Switzerland	0.03	1.00	1.00	0.33	0.38
UK	0.77	0.08	0.25	0.19	0.87
US	0.00	1.00	0.97	1.00	0.01

High access and efficiency

The calibrated dataset for countries which achieve both high access and high efficiency is shown in Table 3.7.

From Table 3.7, the countries achieving a high score for both access and efficiency are Australia, Germany, New Zealand, Norway, Sweden and the UK. In contrast, Canada, France and the US have very low scores.

In calculating possibly necessary conditions, only one term produced a credible statistical fit, ~VOL, which has a consistency of 0.87 and a relevance of 0.71. This term is also credible in terms of the earlier research discussion, so was included in the calculation of the results which follow. However, looking across the data, there is one country with both high access and efficiency that has a high VOL score. Again, Australia proves to be the exception.

The truth table, as with the efficiency results, presented a dilemma in respect of the consistency threshold. If it is produced with the 0.8 consistency threshold benchmark (but which is the same up to 0.874), then it is as shown in Table 3.8.

From Table 3.8, there are two rows included that meet the consistency threshold to be included in the sufficient solution – for New Zealand and the UK, and for Norway and Sweden, so there will be two countries deviant for coverage in the solution – Australia and Germany. If the consistency threshold is reduced to 0.784, then this will add Australia to the solution, having a PRI just below the

Table 3.8: Truth table for high access and efficiency, and health funding

GOV	HEALTHEXP	OOP	VOL	OUT	Consistency	PRI	Cases
0	0	0	1	0	0.516	0.065	CAN
0	0	1	1	0	0.785	0.584	AUS
0	1	1	0	0	0.756	0.000	SWI
0	1	1	1	0	0.450	0.012	US
1	0	0	0	1	0.875	0.698	NZ, UK
1	0	0	1	0	0.509	0.060	FRA
1	1	0	0	0	0.784	0.294	GER, NLD
1	1	1	0	1	0.883	0.622	NOR, SWE

0.6 ideal. If consistency is reduced to 0.783, then this will include Germany and the Netherlands as well as Australia, but the PRI for that row is only 0.294, so that would be a poor decision in terms of that measure. It therefore seems wise to compare the solutions produced with consistency of 0.8, but also 0.784 to see what difference including Australia in the solution term makes.

With a consistency of 0.8, and directional expectations of GOV*~VOL, the combination of which appears in the majority of sufficient high access and efficiency solutions, the intermediate solution was as follows:

Solution	Consistency	PRI	Coverage	Unique coverage	Cases
GOV*HEALTHEXP*OOP *~VOL	0.883	0.622	0.463	0.282	NOR, SWE
GOV*~HEALTHEXP*~OOP *~VOL	0.875	0.698	0.431	0.250	NZ, UK
Solution consistency 0.859, Coverage 0.713					

This solution then has two pathways – both of which combine all four causal factors, and both of which contain the necessary condition ~VOL. The first pathway combines high government spending with high health expenditure, high out-of-pocket expenditure and low voluntary health insurance, covering Norway and Sweden.

The second pathway has high government spending and low voluntary health insurance in common with the first solution pathway, but combines it with low health expenditure and low out-of-pocket expenditure rather than the latter two factors being high, as in the first solution. It covers the cases of New Zealand and the UK.

The conservative solution here is the same as the intermediate one, with the parsimonious solution being simplified to ~HEALTHEXP*~VOL for New Zealand and the UK, or GOV*OOP*~VOL for Norway and Sweden.

This solution term has two cases deviant for coverage, so missing from it – Australia and Germany.

If the consistency of the truth table is reduced to 0.784, with directional expectations of GOV*~VOL, it allows the inclusion of AUS in the intermediate solution term, which changes as follows:

Solution	Consistency	PRI	Coverage	Unique coverage	Cases
~GOV*~HEALTHEXP*OOP	0.794	0.602	0.279	0.126	AUS
GOV*HEALTHEXP*OOP *~VOL	0.883	0.622	0.463	0.282	NOR, SWE
GOV*~HEALTHEXP*~OOP *~VOL	0.875	0.698	0.431	0.210	NZ, UK
Solution consistency 0.821, Coverage 0.839					

There are three solution pathways here, but the second two are identical to ones in the first solution presented earlier.

The first, new pathway combines low government spending with low health expenditure and high out-of-pocket expenditure and covers Australia, adding it to the previous solution, but does not include the necessary condition identified earlier of ~VOL.

The conservative solution is identical to the intermediate solution. The parsimonious solution has an identical first pathway but turns the second pathway into GOV*OOP*~VOL, and the third pathway into ~HEALTHEXP*~VOL.

As such, including AUS in the intermediate solution term reduces consistency from 0.859 to 0.821, but increases coverage from 0.713 to 0.839. It also adds one additional solution pathway to the overall solution (for AUS), but is otherwise identical.

Discussion of results

In terms of high health access, there are two top-level health funding theories that our results can be compared to. The first suggests that high government funding leads to better access to healthcare, as high government funding will mean those who have the least resources should be less likely to be denied the care they need because of the lack of ability to pay for it. The second theory would suggest that it is possible to achieve high healthcare access with higher private (especially out-of-pocket payments, but possibly also voluntary health insurance) because the demand for healthcare will more closely match actual need for it, leading to resources being more effectively deployed. The first theory would suggest that countries such as Norway, Germany and Sweden should have better health access, and the second that Switzerland, the US and Norway (the three highest users of out-of-pocket payments) might achieve better access. Norway has both high government funding and high out-of-pocket payments, and so is of particular interest.

For high access GOV*~VOL was a necessary condition – a mix of high government spending and low voluntary health insurance. This combination appears to be in line with the theory of high government expenditure achieving greater access, while at the same time asking difficult questions about the role of voluntary health insurance in achieving that goal.

However, there was one high access country which was the exception to this condition – Australia. As such that country appears to be the exception in its pattern of health funding, as it was with social determinants as well.

In terms of sufficient conditions, there were two pathways, both based on GOV*~VOL, combined with either high health expenditure in the former or low out-of-pocket payments in the latter. The second pathway contradicts the idea that high out-of-pocket expenditure should lead to better health access because of the improved efficiency of the system.

Australia is also the exception to the sufficient solution, being either a case which is deviant for coverage (in the higher consistency solution), or requiring its own solution pathway if the consistency threshold is reduced to 0.797. Australia, then, continues to be an exceptional case. Rather than having a combination of high government spending and low voluntary health insurance, Australia is the opposite – ~GOV*VOL. Its case therefore again requires greater explanation.

In terms of access, the Commonwealth Fund measure is split into two 'domains'– affordability and timeliness. Australia has a score above zero (so on average, comparatively better than other countries) on both, but does better in terms of timeliness. In affordability, it has negative scores around dental care, but perhaps most importantly in terms of doctor reports of patients struggling to pay for medical bills and high out-of-pocket payments. The Australian system makes extensive use of out-of-pocket payments, and the means by which they are reclaimed, at least to UK eyes, is complex.[1] In general, people appear to be used to the system, and it works effectively, however the Commonwealth Fund affordability measure does seem to indicate that some people are struggling with out-of-pocket payments, perhaps because of the complexity of the system.

In terms of timeliness, Australia scores poorest in relation to waiting times for treatment after diagnosis, pointing to a problem there. Given that the Australian system has a clear split between public and private, and with a great deal of the incentive to take out private health insurance coming from achieving quicker access (as well as access to better facilities), it makes sense to assume that those who have public health insurance coverage only would make up a disproportionate number of those having longer waiting times.

As such, Australia does well in terms of health access, but with its affordability only just falling among those in the highest-performing countries because of its use of out-of-pocket payments, and its weakness in terms of timeliness is likely to be for those with public health insurance only. These aspects are not unique to Australia, but do seem to mark it out in comparison with the other high access countries in the Commonwealth Fund data. Australia achieves high access, but through a different route to other countries achieving the same outcome.

Achieving high efficiency can theoretically have a public or private solution. A highly efficient publicly funded system would be based on economies of scale and scope, as well as the ability to reduce bureaucracy through a unified and coordinated administrative system. However, it may also struggle with diseconomies of scale if too large, and with a bureaucratic detachment if public funding means that money is not spent on patient need, as advocates of public choice theory might suggest. An efficient privately funded system would function through the use of patients driving providers to be more efficient by shopping around for healthcare or for health insurance, and making sure the most efficient providers received the custom. However, it might be subject to problems of information asymmetry, where the public cannot judge whether care is efficient or not as they lack the expertise or knowledge (Arrow, 1963), or efficiency might be reduced where voluntary health insurance is purchased on behalf of the public by intermediaries such as employers.

In terms of efficiency, the necessary conditions are complex as they involve either high government spending or low health expenditure, or high government spending or low out-of-pocket payments. All countries in the sample fit within the first necessary condition, and there is one exception to the latter – Australia again.

The sufficient solutions have two pathways based around GOV*~VOL, and with over four of the six countries achieving high health efficiency. However, those countries can be further split by adding additional factors – either low health expenditure and low out-of-pocket payments (New Zealand and the UK) or high health expenditure and high out-of-pocket payments (Norway and Sweden). These solutions have a common root, but diverge quite significantly in terms of their dynamics, with New Zealand and the UK solution presenting systems based almost entirely around government funding, and being low overall spend, but Norway and Sweden offering high expenditure systems with high out-of-pocket payments.

These solutions offer the possibility of supporting claims about greater efficiency resulting from either public or private funding. New Zealand, Norway, Sweden and the UK have higher levels of efficiency, but within those countries there are two routes, one involving high public funding but low overall expenditure (the UK and New Zealand), and another high public out-of-pocket expenditure, and high overall expenditure (Norway and Sweden).

However, two countries, Australia and Canada, have a solution based around the opposite ~GOV*VOL, and combine it with lower levels of health expenditure. Australia is again proving to be an usual case, but here has the same combination of solution factors as Canada. Canada is a marginal case for being in the high efficiency set of countries, but has consistently good scores across most of the efficiency domains, with the best score of all for doctors' reports of not having to spend time on administrative reporting to government. However, Canada seems to have an issue in relation to patients going to emergency rooms rather than being treated by regular doctors, a measure where it is measured as having the worst score of all the countries in the sample. Australia scores well in every measure of efficiency, and so its overall result is clearly not distorted by outlier scores. What this suggests is that, with the exception of Canada's use of emergency departments instead of regular doctors, both Canada and Australia have genuinely efficient health systems, even though they achieve that goal through very different patterns of health funding to other countries. Theirs is the low health expenditure, low government funding solution to high efficiency.

One country is deviant for coverage from the high efficiency solution, and so is missing from it – Germany. Germany, along with Canada, is overall a marginal high efficiency country. In contrast to Canada, however, Germany's efficiency measure is made up of far more extreme values, with very poor scores for the time doctors spend dealing with insurance claims, and for the time spent on dealing with coverage issues for medications on behalf of patients. However, Germany does well in terms of patient records being available, and in contrast to Canada, patients' use of emergency rooms (rather than people seeing their regular doctors) appears relatively low. Germany's efficiency score then is rather more variable than Canada's, and with two very negative scores in the domain. Germany, then, appears to be risking its reputation of being highly efficient because of the time doctors have to spend when navigating the system. If Germany were able to improve in relation to the bureaucracy which doctors complain of finding so time consuming, it would be able to make a stronger claim to high efficiency. Equally, if we compare Germany with Norway and Sweden, all of which have the pattern GOV*HEALTHEXP*~VOL, and all of which are high efficiency countries, the difference appears to be the higher use of out-of-pocket payments in Norway and Sweden compared to Germany. Perhaps those countries have found a way of doctors spending less time dealing with bureaucracies.

In terms of high access and high efficiency, ~VOL was the single necessary condition, but with Australia again as the exceptional case. The sufficient solution has two pathways based around GOV*~VOL, with the first combining those terms with high health expenditure and high out-of-pocket expenditure (Norway and Sweden), and the second combining it with low health expenditure and low out-of-pocket expenditure (New Zealand and the UK).

These solutions, however, omit Australia and Germany, so these are cases which are deviant for coverage. This is perhaps not surprising given Australia is either an outlier case or deviant for coverage for high access, and Germany is deviant for coverage for high efficiency. The reasons for those cases' deviancy were explored earlier.

Conclusion

There needs to be good access to health systems, otherwise there is the risk of people being ill or injured when they could be helped. Even people who regard personal responsibility as central to their belief systems will accept there is some need for those who cannot afford health services to be able to access them, if only for children and the most vulnerable, but probably for as many people as can reasonably be afforded. Poor access to healthcare raises difficult moral questions about deservingness, but is also plainly economically inefficient – it means that people who could be contributing to the economy and society may be unable to do so because of illness or injury.

In terms of access, theories supporting public funding are supported by the data here, with high government spending and low voluntary health insurance combining in a necessary condition which is at the heart of sufficient solutions which split into a high health expenditure solution, embracing four countries (Germany, the Netherlands, Norway and Sweden), or a low out-of-pocket funding solution, which also has four countries (Germany, the Netherlands, New Zealand and the UK). In either case, high government spending and low voluntary health insurance are at the root of both solutions. However, there is one case that deviates from this pattern – as with solutions in Chapter 2 – Australia.

As well as access being important, health systems need to be efficient as they are so expensive, because efficiency savings (or avoidances of inefficiency) can allow additional healthcare spending, or because it might allow expenditure in other societal areas.

High health efficiency is also compatible with public funding, with high government spending and low voluntary health insurance being at the root of the solutions for four of the six countries achieving high health efficiency, but with Australia (again) along with Canada bucking this trend and having exactly the opposite factors at the heart of their sufficient solution – low government spending and high voluntary health insurance. However, for high health efficiency, there is also room for private funding as the GOV*~VOL sufficient solution splits into two – similarly to that for high access, but more clearly, with a high health funding and high out-of-pocket solution for Norway and Sweden, but a low health funding and low out-of-pocket solution for New Zealand and the UK.

There is therefore a solution based on high government funding, but low overall health expenditure (New Zealand and the UK) and a more mixed solution, including high government and high out-of-pocket funding and high overall health expenditure (Norway and Sweden).

For high access and high efficiency, however, ~VOL is the sole necessary condition. The sufficient condition creates a a similar split of countries as in the solution for sufficient efficiency, with identical mixes of factors for Norway and Sweden on the one hand (GOV*HEALTHEXP*OOP*~VOL) and New Zealand and the UK on the other (GOV*~HEALTHEXP*~OOP*~VOL). However, these sufficient solutions omit Australia (once again) along with Germany.

The countries which therefore score highly for access and efficiency are Norway, Sweden, New Zealand and the UK, which appear in the sufficient solution – but also Australia and Germany, which are deviant for coverage.

Both GOV and VOL repeatedly appear in both necessary and sufficient solutions throughout this chapter, showing that they are perhaps the most important factors in terms of achieving high access and high efficiency, and so they will be carried forward to Chapter 6, where the most important factors found in the book will be considered together.

Australia continues to be the country among our 11 that is most difficult to account for. In terms of health access it is either a case deviant for coverage or a pathway solution on its own if the consistency threshold is lowered. Along with the findings from Chapter 2, it is becoming clear that Australia truly is an exceptional case, but a more detailed exploration of the Commonwealth Fund data shows that Australia genuinely achieves high access and high efficiency.

In contrast, the other case which is deviant for coverage for high access and efficiency, Germany, is more marginal in terms of its efficiency score, and the component parts of its score are extremely variable. That Germany is marginal in that measure, along with the findings from Chapter 2 which found Germany deviant for consistency in terms of high health outcomes, suggests it is an outlier in terms of the data so far analysed in the book, and is not addressing the challenges which are common to the nations here as effectively as might be expected.

The final conclusion in this chapter is a methodological point. In terms of high health access and high health efficiency, there was a balance to be struck between achieving higher consistency for the solution but lower coverage, or reducing the consistency of the solution and achieving a higher coverage. This debate is an important part of QCA, in which the emphasis is on going back and forth between the data and the cases, looking for the best explanations and fits for solutions. Rather than concealing that process, it makes sense to make it as transparent as possible to explain the trade-offs that are being made. In this sense, QCA is a mixed-method research strategy, requiring qualitative judgements about numeric data, and achieving better understanding of the cases as a result.

Case studies

The chapter ends with three more individual country case studies – those of the UK, New Zealand and France.

The United Kingdom

The UK is comprised of four countries, with health being a delegated responsibility in Scotland, Wales and Northern Ireland. England, which has the highest population of the four nations, also houses the central UK government. Despite differences in the post–devolution era, health services across the four nations have a distinctive common character and are generally presented in cross-national comparisons as one, as they are here.

The UK has a National Health Service which aims to provide largely free, comprehensive care to all citizens. The UK has historically been a relatively low spender on healthcare compared to other nations, with some catch-up occurring in the decade 2000–2010. The majority of funding is from general taxes, with a proportion (around 20 per cent) from national insurance payments, which are a payroll tax for employees and employers.

The scope of services offered by the NHS aims to be comprehensive, but can vary in practice in different local areas, and there is no absolute right to receive any particular treatment.

There are co-payments, especially for prescription medicines, but these have substantial exemptions attached to them (with nearly 90 per cent being dispensed free of charge), and are not charged in all the UK nations. It is possible to use NHS services as a private patient to 'jump' the waiting queue or sometimes access improved facilities.

Private health insurance is available in the UK, and is often linked to employment, with around 10 per cent of the population holding voluntary health insurance as a result.

The UK's fuzzy-set scores for funding are as follows:

COUNTRY	GOVCOMP	HEALTHEXP	OOP	VOL
UK	0.77	0.08	0.25	0.36

From this, the UK is a comparatively very low spender on healthcare overall, with the majority of its funding coming from government. The UK makes low use of out-of-pocket payments and its levels of voluntary health insurance are also relatively low.

Long-term care remains a complex and contentious issue, incorporating a high proportion of private expenditure and being variable between the UK nations. The NHS pays for people with advanced needs, but other long-term services are paid for out of pocket or by local authorities, with extensive means and eligibility testing in place. Over three quarters of residential care for the elderly and disabled is provided by the private sector.

The UK's fuzzy-set scores for health expenditure are as follows:

COUNTRY	HEALTHEXP	CUREREHAB	LONG	PREVENT
UK	0.08	0.31	0.59	0.96

The UK has low levels of curative and rehabilitative expenditures, but very high levels of preventative expenditure. Its levels of long-term care are also in the high set.

General practice occupies a traditional gate-keeping role in all four nations, but has been expanded in England to incorporate a commissioning role for local services as well. It is generally not possible to receive specialist care without a GP referral, even for private care. The majority of hospitals are publicly owned, but with some private and not-for-profit facilities available.

England has experimented with commissioning care, first by making primary care organisations responsible (2000s) and then GP commissioning groups (2010s). These experiments built on the 'internal markets' of the 1990s. Scotland, however, has moved to a more partnership and collaborative approach. In practice, the health outcomes of the two nations, however, seem similar so far (Bevan et al, 2014) and seem more linked to changes in levels of funding than to the divergence in organisational forms (Greener, 2018).

In terms of social determinants, the UK's fuzzy-set scores are as follows:

COUNTRY	GINI	BEHAV	EDUC	HEALTHEXP
UK	0.91	0.70	0.82	0.08

The UK has comparatively high income inequality, relatively high levels of behavioural factors (both smoking and drinking), and comparatively high levels of people with pre-secondary education only. When these factors are combined with low overall health expenditures, the UK is unique among the countries here in having a social determinants fuzzy-set configuration which corresponds, according to existing research, with the worst possible combination of factors.

New Zealand

New Zealand's health system is universal and mostly publicly funded through general taxation.

The national government sets the overall budget and also decides the benefit package that will be available through the public system based on a mix of political priorities and health needs. District health boards are responsible for planning purchasing and providing health services locally. The boards must provide the services set by the national government.

There are some co-payments for services, but deductibles are not used. Out-of-pocket payments are nearly 13 per cent of all health funding, and are made to visit GPs (with lower-income patients having fees capped), and for prescription charges (capped at around $3.40 for the first 20 prescriptions per family per year). Private health insurance covers around one third of the population, with it being mostly used to pay for services not covered by the public system, or to help with co-payments, and can also lead to faster access for non-urgent treatment.

New Zealand's health funding fuzzy-set scores are as follows:

COUNTRY	GOV	HEALTHEXP	OOP	VOL
New Zealand	0.82	0.02	0.06	0.52

New Zealand, then, has relatively low levels of health expenditure, proportionally high levels of government funding and it just falls into the high set of voluntary health insurance funding. There are very low levels of out-of-pocket payments.

Long-term care is based on patient needs assessment and means testing, with eligible people receiving comprehensive services either in residential facilities or in their own homes. Individuals with assets over the national threshold pay the cost of their care up to a maximum contribution, and those with assets under the threshold contribute all of their income except for a small personal allowance. District health funding covers differences between payments made by people and the price of their residential care, with in-home care being income tested, and personal care provided free of charge. Home services, in contrast to the rest of the public system, are provided by non-government organisations and there is some experimentation with personal budgets.

Health disparities between Maori and Pacific Island people and the rest of the population remain a significant problem. There is a great deal of data collection and comparison between these different groups showing significant gaps, and district health boards are required to construct health plans to try and deal with them, as well as consulting with Maori and Pacific Island people in the construction of those plans.

New Zealand's social determinants fuzzy-set scores are as follows:

COUNTRY	GINI	BEHAV	EDUC	HEALTHEXP
NZ	0.89	0.37	0.95	0.02

New Zealand has relatively high levels of income inequality, and has very high levels of people with pre-secondary education only. It has relatively low behavioural factors though. When combined with its low levels of overall health expenditures, New Zealand has a pattern of social determinants which is comparable, in fuzzy-set terms, to that of Australia.

France

The French system is funded through mandatory enrolment in a the statutory health insurance system, which is organised around the central government setting a national health strategy and allocated budgets to regional health agencies, which are then responsible for both planning and delivering services. The insurance system is funded through payroll taxes (employer and employee), a national income tax, and through tax levies in some industries and products (tobacco, alcohol, pharmaceutical and private health insurance). The state is responsible for around three quarters of health funding.

Coverage is comprehensive, but there are co-payments, coinsurance and balance billing for physician charges that exceed the fees covered by the public system. Most out-of-pocket spending is for dental and vision services, which have some public funding, but with most providers expecting additional payments (balance-bill). Out-of-pocket expenditures on drugs are increasing, and there are co-payments for primary doctor visits capped per year, with payments to specialist physicians comprising requiring a mix of co-payments and coinsurance. There are also small co-payments for prescription drugs (with coinsurance depending on the judged efficacy of the drug being paid for).

Nearly all French citizens have supplemental insurance to help with out-of-pocket costs. Voluntary health insurance is often sponsored by employers.

The fuzzy-set scores of health funding for France are as follows:

COUNTRY	GOV	HEALTHEXP	OOP	VOL
France	0.76	0.24	0.02	0.93

France spends relatively less on healthcare than other nations in this book and has a distinctive pattern of funding its health system based on high government expenditure, very high voluntary health insurance, but low out-of-pocket payments.

Long-term care is provided in retirement homes and long-term care units, around half of which are public, but with the for-profit sector growing. Statutory health insurance covers care in these institutions, but with housing costs having to be met by families. These costs are often paid for through voluntary health insurance and can be substantial. Statutory health insurance covers some of the revenues for home care, along with a Solidary Fund for Autonomy, which is funded by employers paying their employees' daily wages into it for one day a year. Home care is not means tested. Non-medical home care, however, is means tested, with cash allowances being linked to assessed need.

France's expenditure fuzzy-set scores are as follows:

COUNTRY	HEALTHEXP	CUREREHAB	LONG	PREVENT
FRA	0.24	0.07	0.33	0.05

These scores show France to be a comparatively low spender across all expenditure categories. It is very low for both curative and preventative care, and fairly low for long-term expenditure. If we drill down into these numbers, the curative and rehabilitative score is due to low levels of outpatient expenditure, and with France spending very high levels on medical goods (which include medical devices and pharmaceuticals) rather than the categories of expenditure included here. As such, it is possible that France is accounting for its expenditures in a different way to the other countries in this sample, but there is no way to correct the OECD measures, which are produced in line with a standard set of accounts, so we have little option but to work with the measures.

France's fuzzy-set scores for social determinants are as follows:

COUNTRY	GINI	BEHAV	EDUC	HEALTHEXP
FRA	0.11	0.97	0.90	0.24

France, then, has very low income inequality, but scores very high in terms of behavioural factors (with the highest measures of all the countries here for both smoking and drinking). France also has high numbers of people with pre-secondary education only. This mix is different from the UK, in fuzzy-set terms, in terms of one factor – whereas France has lower levels of income inequality, the UK's are high.

Spending on health

Introduction

Typologies of health system expenditures tend to be based on their degree of publicness (Blank et al, 2018, p 73), or countries are compared on the basis of their total spend on healthcare (Kotlikoff and Hagist, 2005). However, there is still relatively little work which explores different categories of health expenditure and how these contribute to good or bad care, and whether that care, in turn, leads to better or worse health outcomes.

In terms of arguments around levels of expenditure, there is often a general assumption that greater healthcare expenditure allows the purchase of more health services, and that this should lead to better health outcomes. However, this clashes with critical work, perhaps best exemplified by Illich (1977b), suggesting that increased spending on healthcare may itself be detrimental (Blank et al, 2018, p 260), with medicine being portrayed as a 'disabling profession' (Illich, 1977a) that prevents us from trying to find our own sources of well-being. As well as the disabling profession critique, Illich argued that the toxic or dangerous effects of medicine (its 'iatrogenetic' dimension) were not being taken into account, and raised questions that more recent authors (O'Mahony, 2016) have used as a basis for questioning the legitimacy of many medical interventions, which they find fall short of the standards of evidence which medicine aspires to (Stegenga, 2018).

There have been significant debates on the implications of trying to shift expenditure between primary and secondary care, which has been explored both in terms of individual health systems, but also comparatively (Peckham and Exworthy, 2003). There is a general trend towards health systems becoming more 'primary-care led' and of care moving more away from high-cost hospitals into community settings where it can be delivered more responsively (and perhaps more cost-effectively), but conceptual and measurement problems abound of what qualifies as 'primary care' (OECD, 2019), and so, although this debate is an important one, it is not the main focus of this chapter.

When considering what health systems spend their funding on, there are significant challenges involved in trying to balance the acute health needs of people today with expenditure on those with long-term conditions, with changing demography leading to increasing numbers of people with conditions such as asthma or diabetes, which medicine currently often cannot cure, and so which potentially require life time support. At the same time, calls for increased spend on preventative and public health measures (Blank et al, 2018, p 180) require policymakers to either find additional funds or reduce current expenditures – when the returns on such preventative expenditures may not appear for decades.

Despite the substantial work exploring all of these topics, existing research does little to map or categorise countries in relation to their patterns of different health expenditure types. Equally, the links between health expenditures, the measures of care, and health outcomes still remains underexplored territory. This chapter asks what configurations of different categories of healthcare expenditures and their levels exist. What is the relationship between these configurations and the Commonwealth Fund measures of care process and health outcomes?

Without wishing to pre-empt the chapter's results, there is a significant tension in terms of exploring health expenditures in terms of measures of both care and health outcomes – because the two outcome measures have very little in common. This challenge will be referred as the 'care and outcomes paradox' – and will be discussed in greater depth later. It is certainly odd that countries that are assessed in the Commonwealth Fund care measure as high performing seem often to have poor health outcomes.

Health expenditure

The Introduction mapped out some key debates in relation to health expenditures, which this section can explore in greater depth. Whereas there is a great deal of discussion about whether there is a right level of health expenditure, there is less work considering exactly what health expenditures should actually be spent on. However, there are some top-level debates which are important, and are worth exploring in greater depth.

A first view, which makes a great deal of intuitive sense, is that if health expenditures are increased, this will improve healthcare, and this, in turn, should improve health outcomes. As noted in previous chapters, the work of Deaton (2015) and the OECD (2017) seems to at least implicitly support this view, showing the relationship between increased health expenditures and measures such as life expectancy. However, there are strong counter-voices against this view.

Illich (1977a) suggested that contemporary medicine (along with groups such as teachers and lawyers) were 'disabling professions', which interfered with people making their own life choices. In Illich's view, professional groups such as medicine are largely unaccountable to the public, going beyond their expertise to label people, creating demand for their services in the process, and establishing social norms that are inherently political in nature. Instead, Illich emphasised the importance of lived experience, and went further, developing a theory of 'iatrogenesis' (Illich, 1977b), which pointed to the harms done by medicines.

Illich's critical view is not the only one expressing scepticism towards the need to increase health expenditures. Nixon and Ulmann (2006) suggest that increased health expenditures make a difference in terms of infant mortality, but make little difference to life expectancy. Self and Grabowski (2003) report that larger per capita expenditures make little difference to people's health, especially in terms of public health, as people are already economically better off and better educated.

More recent followers in Illich's footsteps have emphasised the importance of medicine being based on personal relationships of care rather than high technology (McCartney, 2012), with critics building on his work on iatrogenesis to highlight significant weakneses in processes for new drug approvals, and the surprisingly unproven status of a great number of commonplace medical treatments (Le Fanu, 2018; O'Mahony, 2019). In this view, healthcare should be much more about making sure people have access to good nutrition, and fostering systems which enable people to live healthy lives, than, in their view, the over-medicalisation that is currently present. This work casts doubt on the intuition that greater funding for healthcare will necessary lead to either better care or better health outcomes.

This book has already shown that the highest spender of all on healthcare, the US, is also ranked last in terms of health outcomes by the Commonwealth Fund. The US also has among the highest preventable mortality measured among the developed countries measured by the OECD (see Chapter 6), with only Estonia and Poland higher. However, it is possible that the US's health expenditure is on the wrong things, and so is an exception to the rule of thumb that higher expenditures lead to the best results.

Moving beyond the debate around levels of health expenditures, at least two more are of importance to this chapter. These are the tension between curative and long-term health expenditures, and between both curative and long-term expenditures, and preventative spending.

Curative versus long-term expenditures

As the demography of societies have changed, life expectancies have increased and lifestyles have changed, then the profiles of disease and illness too have changed. Expenditures on injuries will always be needed, but as people live longer, the prevalence of diseases which increase with age, including several cancers, increase too. As well as this, conditions which used to be called 'chronic' and are now termed 'long-term', such as diabetes and asthma, have become more common. The increase in such long-term conditions, which around one third of people are often estimated to have (Greener, 2008), has led to attempts to increase 'self-management' from patients with such conditions, and to calls for doctors, especially, to recognise the embodied experience of those patients – a demand with at least something in common with the 'disabling professions' critique of Illich outlined earlier. Pressures on government funding in periods of austerity, such as those affecting many developed countries post 2008, mean that attempts to achieve greater self-management from patients can, however, also be seen as an attempt to reduce expenditures rather than increase patient autonomy (Greenhalgh, 2009).

Curative versus preventative

There are also tensions between current health expenditures and those which are designed to change health behaviours, with often substantial gaps between such preventative spend between public health messages designed to reduce smoking rates or obesity levels and any results they might generate. Indeed, many on the political right appear to resent expenditures of this type, suggesting that they patronise people and interfere with their choices (Haidt, 2013; Lakoff, 2016).

Advocates of greater preventative expenditure, in contrast, argue that policymakers should seek to rebalance expenditure between curing people, or preventing disease or illness. At present, every health system here spends vastly more on services whose primary purpose is to cure than on those which seek to engage in health education, promotion and prevention.

There is a difficult tension between expenditure that occurs for people who are ill or injured now, and expenditure that aims to prevent illness or injury in the future. When confronted by people who require healthcare now, there is a responsibility for health services to try and help them. Preventative expenditure, on the other hand, is much more designed to support people in making decisions that will lead to them being disease free or even achieving a higher standard of life, for longer. Where there is a resource-constrained environment, it will be a brave politician who increases spend on preventative care while current health needs are not being fully met – even if that decision is based on the best possible evidence that it will lead to significant gains in the future. Politicians face a dreadful dilemma here – especially when the benefit of preventative care spending may end up appearing in the health outcome measures of their successors because of the often long time lags that are involved. Even if people can be persuaded to lead improved lifestyles today, improvements in health outcomes may not arrive for decades.

As such, exploring the patterns of health expenditures raises questions about the efficacy of increasing health expenditure, between curative expenditures and those designed to manage long-term conditions, and between all items of expenditure designed to address illness and injury today and preventative health expenditures designed to reduce health problems for the future.

The next section explores the data in relation to these expenditure types.

Data and expectations

The OECD data for health expenditure do not use the categories which are familiar in health services discussion between primary, secondary and tertiary care because of significant methodological difficulties in consistently measuring these types of care across health systems (see especially OECD, 2019). However, there are standardised sets of accounts which can address the debates outlined earlier. The OECD categories of expenditure are as follows.

The first OECD category is for curative and rehabilitative expenditure. Curative care is healthcare which is meant to relieve symptoms of illness or injury in order to reduce its severity or protect against it growing worse, or from complications occurring. Curative services focus primarily on health conditions, and rehabilitation services focus on functioning associated with the health condition, aiming to stabilise, improve or restore impaired body functions and structures. These services are those we would often regard as 'acute' in that they address a specific illness or injury which requires immediate treatment. In contrast, but relatedly, rehabilitation services are those that address significant injuries or illnesses that aim to restore bodies after acute illnesses or injuries. In this chapter, this expenditure is labelled 'CURREHAB'.

The second OECD category expenditure is that of long-term care. Long-term care comprises a range of personal care services that are concerned with the primary goal of alleviating pain and suffering and reducing or managing the deterioration of health status in patients with a degree of long-term dependency. Long-term care tends to be less acute than the services provided by curative care, and while it may involve some degree of rehabilitation, it tends to be focused on managing conditions which are either permanent or recurrent.

With people living longer lives, the need to provide long-term care effectively is becoming increasingly important as more and more people have a long-term condition of one kind or another. However, long-term expenditure appears to vary considerably between countries because of difficulties in moving it away from the acute sector (Blank et al, 2018, p 197). Here long-term care is labelled 'LONG'.

The third OECD category of expenditure is that of medical goods, which are medicines and other goods which are part of a package of services with a preventative, curative, rehabilitative or long-term care purpose. Because medical goods can fit with curative, long-term or preventative care, they are not included in the analysis here. This decision was also taken because of the risk of increasing causal categories to a point where 'limited diversity' reached a point where large numbers of possible combinations of factors did not have actual cases present – and with 10 cases (New Zealand do not comply with the OECD system of health accounts so cannot be included in this chapter), this is an important consideration.

The fourth OECD health expenditure category is that of preventative care. This consists of expenditure that aims to reduce the number or severity of injuries and diseases, and is based on a health promotion strategy that involves a process to improve health through the control of some of its immediate determinants. Here, preventable care expenditure is labelled 'PREVENT'.

The next OECD categorisation of expenditure is that of governance and health system and financing administration. This expenditure is concerned with spending on the health system rather than with the provision of healthcare directly, on services that direct support health system functioning, and as such does not contribute to care directly is not included here.

The OECD has an additional category of expenditure that is not included in analysis here. Spend on ancillary services is concerned with services the purpose of which is diagnosis and monitoring, and which, according to the OECD 'do not, therefore, have a purpose in themselves'. As such, again, it is not included here.

Table 4.1: Health expenditure calibrated dataset for 10 countries

COUNTRY	HEALTHEXP	CUREREHAB	LONG	PREVENT
AUS	0.30	0.98	0.02	0.03
CAN	0.33	0.09	0.42	0.98
FRA	0.24	0.07	0.33	0.05
GER	0.83	0.28	0.35	0.57
NLD	0.76	0.08	0.93	0.87
NOR	0.99	0.21	0.97	0.24
SWE	0.81	0.37	0.94	0.68
SWI	1.00	0.69	0.64	0.24
UK	0.08	0.31	0.59	0.96
US	1.00	0.97	0.06	0.61

From this review, the issue of how levels of health expenditure vary with types is an important one with relatively little research, and so the 'HEALTHEXP' measure which is present in the previous two chapters is also included here. That resulted in the calibrated data set shown in Table 4.1.

In Table 4.1, HEALTHEXP represents health expenditure, CUREREHAB is 'curative and rehabilitative' expenditure, LONG is long-term expenditure, and 'PREVENT' is preventative health expenditure.

From Table 4.1, the US and Australia have the highest expenditures on curative and rehabilitative care by some margin, with the US also being a high spender on preventative care but very low on long-term care, and with Australia very low for both. The highest spenders on long-term care are the Netherlands, Norway and Sweden, with the Netherlands and Switzerland also spending highly on preventative care. The highest spenders on preventative care are Canada, the UK and the Netherlands, with Canada being low spenders in all other categories, and the UK falling just into the high set of spenders for long-term care, but low on curative and rehabilitative expenditures.

The configuration of the cases can be summarised in terms of the set in which causal combinations score over 1.0 as shown in Table 4.2.

As such, there is less in common between countries in terms of expenditures than for social determinants or health funding, with only one pattern of causal combinations in common – between the Netherlands and Sweden.

Table 4.2: Health expenditure truth table combinations

HEALTHEXP	CURREHAB	LONG	PREVENT	CASES
0	0	0	0	FRA
0	0	0	1	CAN
0	0	1	1	UK
0	1	0	0	AUS
1	0	0	1	GER
1	0	1	0	NOR
1	0	1	1	NLD, SWE
1	1	0	1	US
1	1	1	0	SWI

In terms of directional expectations, for high care a combination of high curative and rehabilitative and high long-term care were included, on the grounds that those two areas of expenditure were most likely to improve care for those receiving it now.

For health outcomes, a combination of curative and rehabilitative, long-term care and preventative care were included on the grounds that, as well as improving health outcomes now, preventative care expenditure should also improve it in the future.

The calibrated scores for health expenditure causal factors and care are as shown in Table 4.3.

From Table 4.3 the countries with high care scores are the UK, Australia, the Netherlands, the US and Canada. Low care scores appear for Switzerland, Germany, France, Norway and Sweden. The profiles of countries achieving high and low scores seems rather different to previous chapters – a theme to which we will return later.

High care score results

In considering necessary conditions, the combination of high curative and rehabilitative expenditure or preventative expenditure (CURREHAB+PREVENT) had a consistency of 0.99 and a coverage of 0.61, also fitting with our theoretical expectations that good care could be the result of either of these items of expenditure. This combination is included as a necessary condition the analysis.

The necessary condition has a logical OR, with Canada, the Netherlands, the UK and the US having high PREVENT, and Australia and the US have high CURREHAB.

Table 4.3: Calibrated health expenditure and high care scores

COUNTRY	HEALTHEXP	CUREREHAB	LONG	PREVENT	CARE
AUS	0.30	0.98	0.02	0.03	0.87
CAN	0.33	0.09	0.42	0.98	0.68
FRA	0.24	0.07	0.33	0.05	0.15
GER	0.83	0.28	0.35	0.57	0.38
NLD	0.76	0.08	0.93	0.87	0.81
NOR	0.99	0.21	0.97	0.24	0.07
SWE	0.81	0.37	0.94	0.68	0.03
SWI	1.00	0.69	0.64	0.24	0.47
UK	0.08	0.31	0.59	0.96	0.94
US	1.00	0.97	0.06	0.61	0.76

The truth table (Table 4.4) was constructed with a consistency threshold of 0.8 but works up to 0.903. Germany falls within this consistency threshold, but has a low PRI score (0.104), so was excluded through the use of a PRI threshold of 0.5 being added to preventative a simultaneous subset relation in which Germany appeared in both the high and low care scores solution.

Table 4.4 led to the calculation of the intermediate sufficient solution with directional expectations of CUREHAB*LONG.

Solution	Consistency	PRI	Coverage	Unique coverage	Cases
~HEALTHEXP*CUREREHAB *~PREVENT	0.873	0.779	0.217	0.135	AUS
~HEALTHEXP*~CUREREHAB *PREVENT	0.921	0.864	0.365	0.263	CAN, UK
HEALTHEXP*CUREREHAB *~LONG*PREVENT	0.980	0.927	0.294	0.192	US
Solution consistency 0.957, Coverage 0.694					

This solution produces no cases deviant for consistency, but the Netherlands is deviant for coverage so missing from the solution.

Another immediate observation is that the solution sets include two countries (Canada and the US) that have not made many appearances in high solution sets in the book so far – with Canada appearing for high efficiency only, and the US in no high sets at all. As such, the

Table 4.4: Truth table for high care scores and health expenditure

HEALTHEXP	CURREHAB	LONG	PREVENT	OUT	CONSISTENCY	PRI	CASES
0	0	0	0	0	0.471	0.000	FRA
0	0	0	1	1	0.977	0.952	CAN
0	0	1	1	1	0.904	0.808	UK
0	1	0	0	1	0.973	0.949	AUS
1	0	0	1	0	0.846	0.104	GER
1	0	1	0	0	0.517	0.000	NOR
1	0	1	1	0	0.719	0.436	NLD, SWE
1	1	0	1	1	0.980	0.927	US
1	1	1	0	0	0.657	0.000	SWI

countries in the high care solution set are not typical in terms of the solutions so far generated in the book.

The conservative solution is identical, and one of the possible parsimonious solutions is also identical, suggesting there is a high degree of convergence upon the solution offered earlier.

The solutions suggest that there are three pathways to a high care score.

The first pathway combines low health expenditure with high curative expenditure and low preventative expenditure. It covers the case of Australia only. It includes the curative necessary condition.

The second pathway combines low health expenditure with low curative expenditure but high preventative expenditure. It covers the cases of Canada and the UK. It includes the preventative necessary condition.

The third pathway combines high health expenditure with high curative expenditure and high preventative expenditure, but low long-term expenditure. It covers the case of the US. It includes both necessary conditions.

As such, there is something of a mixed solution set here. The solution with the highest coverage and highest unique coverage (pathway 2) has only high preventative care that fits with existing theory and research, with the other two factors (low health expenditure and low curative expenditure) being challenging, to say the least, in terms of our directional expectations, but which do have some links to the claims of Illich and those who have succeeded him.

Results: high health outcomes

For high health outcomes, the calibrated dataset is as shown in Table 4.5.

From Table 4.5 the countries with high outcomes scores are Australia, Sweden, Norway, Switzerland, France and the Netherlands, whereas those with low scores are Germany, Canada, the UK and the US.

In calculating necessary conditions, ~HEALTHEXP+LONG had a consistency of 0.919 and a relevance of 0.730. It offered a dilemma in that lower health expenditure is clearly incompatible with both OECD (2017) and Deaton's (2015) research, but the very high consistency and relevance suggested that the solution term needed to be treated seriously. Of the countries with high health outcomes, ~HEALTHEXP applies to Australia and France, whereas LONG applies to the Netherlands, Norway, Sweden and Switzerland. The two necessary conditions here then are mutually exclusive. The sufficient solutions that follow were generated including their combination as necessary, and to explore the implications of that choice.

The truth table (Table 4.6) was produced with a consistency of 0.8, but produces the same result up to 0.848.

Table 4.6 offered no real dilemmas around consistency, and the intermediate sufficient solution was calculated with directional expectations of CURREHAB*LONG*PREVENT.

Table 4.5: Calibrated dataset for high health outcomes and health expenditure

COUNTRY	HEALTHEXP	CUREREHAB	LONG	PREVENT	HEALTH OUTCOMES
AUS	0.30	0.98	0.02	0.03	0.95
CAN	0.33	0.09	0.42	0.98	0.19
FRA	0.24	0.07	0.33	0.05	0.76
GER	0.83	0.28	0.35	0.57	0.32
NLD	0.76	0.08	0.93	0.87	0.54
NOR	0.99	0.21	0.97	0.24	0.89
SWE	0.81	0.37	0.94	0.68	0.94
SWI	1.00	0.69	0.64	0.24	0.82
UK	0.08	0.31	0.59	0.96	0.07
US	1.00	0.97	0.06	0.61	0.04

Table 4.6: Truth table for high health outcomes and health expenditure

HEALTHEXP	CUREHEAB	LONG	PREVENT	OUT	CONSISTENCY	PRI	CASES
0	0	0	0	1	1.000	1.000	FRA
0	0	0	1	0	0.461	0.000	CAN
0	0	1	1	0	0.548	0.145	UK
0	1	0	0	1	1.000	1.000	AUS
1	0	0	1	0	0.722	0.133	GER
1	0	1	0	1	0.985	0.970	NOR
1	0	1	1	1	0.849	0.669	NLD, SWE
1	1	0	1	0	0.619	0.097	US
1	1	1	0	1	0.989	0.977	SWI

Solution	Consistency	PRI	Coverage	Unique coverage	Cases
HEALTHEXP*LONG	0.880	0.801	0.678	0.565	NLD, NOR, SWE, SWI
~HEALTHEXP*~LONG *~PREVENT	1.000	1.000	0.317	0.203	AUS, FRA
Solution consistency 0.905, Coverage 0.881					

This solution has both high consistency and high coverage, with no cases deviant for either consistency or coverage.

The first solution pathway combines high health expenditure with high long-term expenditure, and covers Norway, the Netherlands, Sweden and Switzerland. It includes the LONG necessary condition.

The second pathway combines low health expenditure with low long-term expenditure and low preventative expenditure, and covers France and Australia. It includes the ~HEALTHEXP necessary condition.

The conservative solution is the same for Australia and France but splits the first solution pathway into solutions for the Netherlands, Norway and Sweden (HEALTHEXP★~CURREHAB★LONG) and for Norway and Switzerland (HEALTHEXP★LONG★~PREVENT). This increases the consistency of the solution to 0.914, but reduces coverage to 0.832. The parsimonious solution is identical to the intermediate solution.

Results: high care score and high outcomes score

The calibrated scores for high care and high outcomes – which following fuzzy-set logic take the lower score of the two – are shown in Table 4.7.

From Table 4.7, the countries with high care and outcomes scores are Australia and the Netherlands only. Switzerland falls just short because of that country's care score (outcomes are scored at 0.82). The lack of countries achieving scores in both of these elements demonstrates the apparent paradox between care and health outcomes – it makes sense for these two scores to be strongly related, as good care should lead to good health outcomes, and yet only two countries achieve high scores in both categories.

There were no necessary conditions with a relevancy score approaching 0.6, so the decision was taken not to include them in the calculations that follow.

The truth table (Table 4.8) was generated with a consistency threshold of 0.8, but works up to 0.972 as there is one case only (Australia) with a consistency at a threshold which could be included in a sufficient solution. This is because the second country with a high care and outcomes score, the Netherlands, has the same patterns of causal factors as Sweden, which we can see falls at the bottom end of the outcome set because of its very poor care score.

Table 4.7: Calibrated dataset for high care and health outcomes and health expenditure for 10 countries

COUNTRY	HEALTHEXP	CUREREHAB	LONG	PREVENT	CARE AND OUTCOMES
AUS	0.30	0.98	0.02	0.03	0.87
CAN	0.33	0.09	0.42	0.98	0.19
FRA	0.24	0.07	0.33	0.05	0.15
GER	0.83	0.28	0.35	0.57	0.32
NLD	0.76	0.08	0.93	0.87	0.54
NOR	0.99	0.21	0.97	0.24	0.07
SWE	0.81	0.37	0.94	0.68	0.03
SWI	1.00	0.69	0.64	0.24	0.47
UK	0.08	0.31	0.59	0.96	0.07
US	1.00	0.97	0.06	0.61	0.04

Table 4.8: Truth table for high care and health outcomes, and health expenditure

HEALTHEXP	CUREREHAB	LONG	PREVENT	OUT	CONSISTENCY	PRI	CASES
0	0	0	0	0	0.471	0.000	FRA
0	0	0	1	0	0.439	0.000	CAN
0	0	1	1	0	0.453	0.000	UK
0	1	0	0	1	0.973	0.949	AUS
1	0	0	1	0	0.701	0.000	GER
1	0	1	0	0	0.502	0.000	NOR
1	0	1	1	0	0.568	0.059	NLD,SWE
1	1	0	1	0	0.599	0.000	US
1	1	1	0	0	0.646	0.000	SWI

The sufficient solution for Table 4.8, then, can only include one country, and does so. The actual solution depends on assumptions about counterfactuals as there is only one case to include. The parsimonious solution is ~HEALTHEXP*CURREHAB with a consistency of 0.747, and the conservative solution simply reproduces all of Australia's causal factors with a consistency of 0.973. Intermediate solutions vary depending on directional expectations, but including CUREREHAB*PREVENT produces ~HEALTHEXP*CURREHAB*~LONG as a solution with a consistency of 0.812. The care and outcomes paradox leads to a sufficient solution which applies to one country only – Australia. This means that the Netherlands, as noted earlier, is deviant for coverage as it appears on the same truth table line as Sweden, and so has a consistency for the outcome of 0.568.

Discussion of results

The solutions for high care are unusual in that they include countries that have not been central to the high outcome solutions in Chapters 2 and 3. The countries which are in the high care solution are Australia (which has been identified as an outlier case in Chapters 2 and 3), Canada (which has only appeared with Australia in the solution for high efficiency) and the US (which has scored poorly in terms of health outcomes, equity, access and efficiency). The UK has appeared frequently in previous solutions, scoring highly for health equity, access and efficiency, and here has the same pattern of factors as Canada, whereas for health funding it had the same pattern of factors as New Zealand. The Netherlands is a case deviant for coverage.

The countries achieving high care scores are much more mixed than has been the case in previous chapters, and this should give pause for thought. If Canada and the US especially are providing such good care, why are they not scoring highly in other health outcome measures as well? This seems to suggest that, although care scores are important, they need to be treated cautiously.

The combination of CURREHAB+PREVENT (curative and rehabilitative expenditure, or preventative expenditure) was a necessary condition for high care. There were three sufficient solutions, with the solution for Australia and the US being unique to that country, and with CAN and the US being covered by a combination of ~HEALTHEXP*~CURREHAB*PREVENT. Two of these solution terms, ~HEALTH*~CURREHAB, were in common with the sufficient solution for Australia as well, indicating this combination of factors is at the root of four of the five countries with high care. This combination suggests that the countries with the highest care scores are those that spend less on healthcare overall, spend less on curative and rehabilitative expenditure, but have higher spends on preventative care. This solution is partially explained by preventative care being one of the four key domains in the Commonwealth Fund care process measure, and so some co-variance might be expected. However, because there are so many other care process domains making up the final score, this relationship should be minimal. It is not clear why lower health expenditure, or lower curative and rehabilitative expenditure, should be linked to high achievement in these measures of care. There is an argument, in line with research stemming from Illich (1977a, b) that this pattern might lead to better care, but the countries which were graded as producing high-quality care were so different to those producing other high outcome measures that this conclusion does not appear entirely credible. This casts further doubt on the Commonwealth Fund care measure.

If the care process measure has proven complex, the link between health expenditure and health outcomes is less problematic.

For high health outcomes there is a necessary condition of ~HEALTHEXP+LONG. At first glance this combination appears confusing as high long-term expenditure could be seen as having a theoretical link to better health outcomes, given the increasing growth of long-term conditions and the importance of supporting people with those conditions. However, low health expenditure is less obvious – especially given the prevalence of high health outcomes across the solutions of Chapter 2, and in key pathways in Chapter 3. However, the two terms comprising the necessary condition are mutually exclusive, with ~HEALTHEXP applying to Australia and France, whereas LONG applies to four countries with also have HEALTHEXP as part of their solution term. The highest coverage pathway for high health outcomes is HEALTHEXP*LONG and covers four countries – it therefore accounts for the inclusion of LONG as a necessary factor, but HEALTHEXP is the exact opposite of ~HEALTHEXP in the necessary condition (but is still consistent with it, because the necessary condition was ~HEALTHEXP+LONG). The second sufficient pathway, however, which covers AUS and FRA, is ~HEALTHEXP*~LONG*~PREVENT, and so has two conditions that are in the opposite direction compared to those of the first pathway, which are then combined with low preventative expenditure. Australia is again an exceptional case – here with France.

Whereas HEALTHEXP*LONG fits with existing theory and research fairly straightforwardly – with high health outcomes being the result of a combination of higher health expenditures and higher spends on long-term care, the solution for Australia (and France) is again a less obvious combination of causal factors, suggesting that high health outcomes can be achieved through an entirely different route than that which has been taken by the Netherlands, Norway, Sweden and Switzerland.

There are only two countries with both high care and high health outcomes – Australia and the Netherlands – and only Australia appears in the sufficient solution. This solution makes clear what might be termed the 'care and outcomes' paradox in the Commonwealth Fund data – that the countries achieving high care scores are very often not the same as those which achieve high health outcomes. This is true for the Commonwealth Fund data in 2017, but also for the report in 2014 (Davis et al, 2014), suggesting the result in 2017 was not a fluke. Why might the 'care and outcomes' paradox exist?

A first explanation is that there are other factors (such as the social determinants of health) which are important in explaining health outcomes. In that view, care is only one aspect of a health system, and perhaps, on the basis of the results here, not even the most significant one in terms of producing good health outcomes. This view makes a great deal of sense. At the same time, it does seem odd that the countries which score highly for care are also often those that do so badly in terms of health outcomes. Even if the care provided by a health system is not the only factor leading to health outcomes, that the countries graded as having a good care process seem so unrelated to those achieving high health outcomes appears a strange result.

Another explanation is that strong care scores today may take time to develop high health outcomes – that there might be a lag before good care turns into results. However, the main problem here is that the Commonwealth Fund has reported on care going back to 2004. In that time the method of calculating care results has evolved rather than changed outright, but across those years the UK, for example, has scored consistently well in terms of care (with perhaps the exception of the patient-centredness measure), and yet its health outcome measures are poor. If there is a lag in results, it is taking the health outcome measure a long time to adjust.

A third explanation is that the care measures are accurate, but the health outcome measures are problematic. However, the same countries that achieve strong health outcomes also appear in solutions based on high access, efficiency and equity, and so consistently score highly across those countries. Equally, the health outcomes measure, being based on robust measures such as life expectancy, preventable mortality (see also Chapter 6), and disease-specific health outcomes, is perhaps one of the strongest measures in the whole dataset.

As such, the care-outcomes paradox appears to be resolved by suggesting that the Commonwealth Fund measure of care, although it is clear and transparent, is not capturing something significant about care, and seems less reliable than the other measures in the dataset.

Conclusion

This chapter is an odd one in the wider context of the book as it has called the Commonwealth Fund 'care process' outcome measure into question because of the disconnect between it, and the 'health outcomes' measure. This disconnect was referred to as the 'care-outcomes' paradox, and reasons for its existence have been suggested in the earlier discussion. In the end, however, the health outcomes measure is based on a clear set of objective indicators, and the high care outcome measure includes countries where there are clear issues with care being offered. As such, it seems clear that the health outcomes measure is the more reliable of the two.

The health outcomes sufficient solution is highly consistent. It is based on two pathways, one of which includes countries which perform strongly in terms of other outcome measures in the book. The necessary condition for high health outcomes (~HEALTHEXP+LONG) is perhaps initially surprising, until the sufficient solution makes clear that the first term relates to Australia (with France), and with

Australia being an outlying case for much of the book, whereas the Netherlands, Norway, Sweden and Switzerland have the combination of HEALTHEXP*LONG, which is much more in line with our theoretical expectations. This solution, in line with that for social determinants, suggests that high health expenditures, in conjunction with high long-term expenditure, are central to the achievement of high health outcomes. The importance of long-term health expenditures means that factor will be carried forward to Chapter 6 as a key factor for consideration there (as levels of health expenditure were already carried forward from Chapter 2 they need not be included again), when further work comparing health systems will be carried out.

The appearance of Australia in what might be considered 'alternative' or 'minority' solution pathways continued in this chapter, so it remains an intriguing case. The key question it asks, perhaps, is whether Australia offers a pattern of causal factors from which other countries can learn, or whether it is too different from other countries for them to be able to learn lessons from it.

Case studies

The chapter ends with the book's two final case studies –for Canada and the USA. Canada and the USA went from having two of the most similar health systems in the world in the 1920s, onto sharply divergent paths afterwards (Tuohy, 1999). Canada moved to a public funding model, the US to a system dominated by private sources of funding.

Canada

Canada has a decentralised, universal, public-funded health system (Medicare). The health system is funded and administered by the 13 provinces and territories, each having its own insurance plan, topped up with funding from the central government, but with the central government giving all citizens all medically necessary hospital and doctor care free at the point of use. Public sources make up around seven tenths of all funding, with private making up the difference.

Many people face charges for prescription drugs (out of hospital), vision and dental care, but with particular groups facing exemptions (typically those on social assistance or of retirement age). Around two thirds of Canadians take out private health insurance to cover them against these charges, but with the vast majority being paid for by employers or other forms of group contracts.

Canada's fuzzy-set pattern of health funding is as follows:

COUNTRY	GOV	HEALTHEXP	OOP	VOL
Canada	0.20	0.33	0.36	0.95

As such Canada is a relatively low spender on healthcare, as well as making comparatively little use of government and out-of-pocket funding. However, its levels of voluntary health insurance are very high.

Doctors are not allowed to charge prices above the negotiated fee schedule, so there is, in effect, no-costsharing for doctor, diagnostic or hospital services. Hospitals are a mix of public and private (predominantly not-for-profit) organisations, but with most provinces and territories having public ownership. Budgets are negotiated with the provincial ministry of health.

Long-term care is provided in non-hospital facilities and is generally not covered by Medicare. However, the services are funded at the provincial level through general taxation, but with significantly different provision between provinces. Government funds personal and nursing care in long-term facilities, with some supplements to help cover room and board costs. Many provinces require co-payments. Eligibility for home-based care is via needs assessment, with some provinces also including means testing.

Canada's fuzzy-set pattern of health expenditure is:

COUNTRY	HEALTHEXP	CUREREHAB	LONG	PREVENT
CAN	0.33	0.09	0.42	0.98

As such, Canada has comparatively very high preventative care expenditures, but very low curative and rehabilitative expenditure. Its level of long-term expenditure is just below the crossover threshold but places it in the low set of countries.

There are significant gaps between indigenous and non-indigenous Canadians, with a central federal budget attempting to help address the problem. Strategies are in place, but as in many other countries sharing the same challenges, progress appears to be slow. Canada's social determinants fuzzy-set scores are:

COUNTRY	GINI	BEHAV	EDUC	HEALTHEXP
CAN	0.28	0.23	0.04	0.33

As such, Canada has low income inequality, low behavioural factors and very low number of people with low levels of education – with the exception of the overall expenditure level, which is lower than ideal, and so has a very strong combination of social determinant factors.

The United States

The US has possibly the most complex health system in the world. The most significant innovation in recent years, the ACA, became law in 2010, but around 8 per cent of people remain uninsured for healthcare, and it was a repeated goal of the Trump presidency to repeal 'Obamacare'.

The US does not have universal health insurance coverage and is financed through a mix of private, public and not-for-profit insurers and supplied by an equally diverse range of healthcare providers. The government Medicare programme funds are for adults aged 65 or over, with Medicaid attempting to support those on low incomes, but with decisions about coverage often delegated to state level and strongly means tested. Attempts to introduce universal health coverage or insurance were repeatedly defeated through the 20th century, and have resulted in the vast literature exploring the ideological, institutional and political barriers to changing the US health system (Wilsford, 1994; Skocpol, 1997; Gordon, 2009; Beland and Waddan, 2012; Starr, 2013).

The Patient Protection and Affordable Care Act, implemented in 2014, was designed to make health insurance available to all Americans at an affordable rate, but also required them to obtain valid health insurance or pay a penalty, although the penalty was later removed. It was organised around creating health insurance marketplaces or exchanges, which offered premium subsidies for those who were eligible not to pay full costs. The ACA did reduce the number of uninsured people from around 20 per cent of the working-age population to around 12 per cent, but that still leaves a huge number of people without reliable health coverage.

Public funding is around 45 per cent of total health spending, by far the lowest of the countries included in this book. Medicare and Medicaid are largely tax funded. In OECD statistics, the introduction of the ACA significantly increased the take-up of health insurance, but as there are no fines attached to not taking out insurance, categorising the sources of funding in the current US system is extremely difficult.

Private health insurance accounts for around one third of all funding but underpins funding for the health system for around two thirds of Americans. The majority of the funding is employer sponsored, with around one third of Americans making use of the exchanges introduced by the ACA to purchase a private Medicaid plan.

America has by far the most expensive healthcare system in the world, having a combination of a public system which spends almost as much (as a proportion of GDP) as the total health expenditure of countries at the lowest end of our sample here, but has in addition a private health system that is at least as big again. Costs and coverage have been the two major issues that policymakers have attempted to overcome in reform efforts, but, as noted earlier, they have faced massive political and institutional barriers to achieving change. The US's health funding fuzzy-set scores are as follows:

COUNTRY	GOV	HEALTHEXP	OOP	VOL
US	0.00	1.00	0.97	1.00

The US then, is a country of extremes in terms of its health funding, being at the extreme high end for overall health expenditure, in its use of out-of-pocket payments and voluntary health insurance, but at the extreme low end for government and compulsory health insurance.

There is no nationally defined health benefit package, with coverage varying significantly depending on insurance type. States vary their Medicaid packages subject to federal minimum requirements.

Individuals finance around 30 per cent of their healthcare costs themselves, with out-of-pocket payments representing about 10 per cent of total health expenditures. There is extensive use of deductibles. Healthcare costs are one of the leading causes of bankruptcy in the US.

There is a federal law that hospitals must treat patients requiring emergency care, regardless of ability to pay or insurance status. Private providers are therefore also a significant source of charitable care.

There is no universal coverage of long-term care services, but public funding covers around 70 per cent of total spending on services, most of which are funded through Medicaid. The public long-term insurance element of the ACA, designed to address problems with the long-term care system, was repealed in 2013. The US's health expenditure fuzzy-set scores are:

COUNTRY	HEALTHEXP	CUREREHAB	LONG	PREVENT
US	1.00	0.97	0.06	0.61

These sets of figures again show the US as representing extremes in three of the four categories, with health expenditure, and curative and rehabilitative expenditure very high, long-term care very low, and preventative care in the high set, but not at the same extreme.

There are significant health gaps between different groups in the US, with African Americans, American Indians, Alaska Natives and Pacific Islanders, along with Hispanics and Asian Americans, receiving poorer care than white Americans according to most quality measures.

The ACA required non-profit hospitals to carry out community needs assessments, and there are specific health services designed to address the needs of American Indians and Alaska Natives. However, in all, the US faces significant challenges in terms of health inequalities, and the US as a whole has the worst health outcomes of all the countries in this book. The US's social determinant fuzzy-set scores are:

COUNTRY	GINI	BEHAV	EDUC	HEALTHEXP
US	0.99	0.12	0.06	1.00

Once again, the US's fuzzy social determinants fuzzy-set scores put it at extremes. Both its income inequality and health expenditure scores are extremely high, whereas for behavioural factors and levels of pre-secondary education only, its scores are very low.

5

COVID-19

Introduction

This chapter utilises the same method as the rest of the book (QCA) but with a different dataset. During the book's writing, the COVID-19 pandemic began and spread across the world. This gave me two options – I could ignore it, as the pandemic was not in the original book proposal, or I could incorporate it, and see how different health systems had responded to the challenge that it offered. I have decided on the latter, but of course any analysis I can offer is limited in that, at the time of writing, the pandemic is far from over. This has resulted in some methodological choices about what I can and cannot write about, but I hope that the chapter offers an insight into the 'first wave' of the pandemic and so makes a contribution to the comparative analysis of health systems.

Understanding why some countries were more successful than others in responding to the pandemic in its first wave – with the analysis here running up to mid July 2020 – gives important insights into the relative importance of the structural influences which are now known to be important in containing the virus, as well as giving an opportunity to assess the success (or otherwise) of different countries' COVID-19 testing regimes.

Comparative studies have the potential to bring insight into how COVID-19 risk factors and testing regimes interrelate, but there are significant data limitations in terms of what can and cannot be measured in a robust way at the time of writing. This necessarily means some compromises have to be made. It is clear that policy responses such as the extent and timing of lockdown restrictions, hygiene measures, border controls, availability of protective equipment, and COVID-19 testing regimes, all have important roles to play. But achieving robust comparative data capturing these factors remains extremely difficult.

It is clear, however, that several important COVID-19 risk factors can be measured. Research over the last six months has shown clearly that older people are more susceptible to the virus and that there are increased risks through obesity (Goldacre and OpenSAFELY Collaborative, 2020). Both of these factors have pre-existing OECD datasets available, and it make sense to consider whether countries with higher levels in these two factors have also had higher COVID-19 mortality as a result. Beyond age and obesity, social deprivation increasingly appears to have a strong link to COVID-19 mortality, and this may have strong intersectional links with minority ethnic groups, which tend to be disproportionately represented in socially deprived groups (Kirby, 2020).

COVID-19 represents the most significant public health challenge developed nations have faced in the modern era. It has prompted a massive research and policy response, with the race for a vaccine being a massive international challenge, but there is clearly a need to attempt to systematise and work through what has emerged in the early months of the pandemic in terms of contextual factors and the policy response to see what can be learned. Work by the Economist Intelligence Unit (Economist Intelligence Unit, 2020) in June 2020 brought together data for OECD nations, comparing a range of risk factors and policy response variables to grade how well countries have dealt with the virus in its early months. Expanding on that data, providing a rigorous analysis using QCA, and exploring the solutions for patterns (as in previous chapters) gives a means of exploring 'first-wave' COVID-19 response, and this chapter aims to achieve this.

Data and calibration

As noted earlier, there are limitations on the data that can be included in a comparative study of both contextual factors and policy response to COVID. Two factors are straightforward – the OECD have robust measures for the proportion of the population categorised as 'elderly' (65+), and this can be included as a first factor. The OECD also collect comparative obesity statistics, which, although not as complete as those for the proportion of elderly, are available for most countries. A third risk factor identified earlier was in relation to social deprivation, which is difficult to comparatively measure directly, but in common with the rest of the book, the GINI income coefficient will be taken as it is generally used as a proxy measure and is used in a great deal of comparative research in developed countries for the purpose of giving an indicator of the breadth of deprivation likely to be present.

Including population density initially sounds like a good idea because of the virus spreading rapidly in crowds (especially indoors), but national population density statistics struggle to capture the size of countries such as the US, or the concentration of cities in particular areas, such as in Australia. Although statistics are available, this factor will not therefore be included here.

The Economist Intelligence Unit's report makes use of a factor not generally included in COVID-19 research, the World Bank international arrivals per overall population, to attempt to assess the openness of countries to international visitors. This measure gives an indication of the initial openness of countries to cross-border spread, and while having the shortcoming of not capturing the situation post lockdown in all nations, does give an indicator in the first months of the pandemic of the extent to which countries were open to international visitors.

In terms of policy response, governments have engaged in a wide range of different activities, and there are emergent indexes[1] which attempt to assess the severity of lockdown measures. However, these indexes are still very new, and perhaps struggle to capture the differences between contexts – a country which is an established tourist destination and with lots of international trade and extensive land borders is in a very different position to countries with none of those features.

One key factor which is available for a large number (but not all) of countries is the number of COVID-19 tests that have been carried out. Given the advice of the World Health Organization from the beginning of the pandemic to 'test, test, test' (WHO, 2020), the ability of governments to put in place a robust testing regime is a reasonable proxy for the effectiveness of their response. Here, tests are measured in relation to population size to make the data comparable.

In terms of measuring the effectiveness of the COVID-19 response, excess mortality is probably the best indictor as it takes into account not only deaths directly linked to COVID, but other COVID-19 deaths which have occurred for which tests may not have been carried out, as well as assessing the indirect effects on mortality of other health challenges that may have been exacerbated by the pandemic. However, again, robust comparative measures of excess mortality are still not in place beyond a very few countries. There are, however, comparative mortality statistics for deaths directly attributed to COVID available, which, although they have differences in methodology, do give an indication of which countries have relatively low and high mortality, so making it possible to derive fuzzy-sets from the data.

Two more things remain in terms of the construction of the initial dataset. First, as well as including tests per population, a measure of tests per COVID-19 case (TESTCASE) was constructed on the grounds that this would scale the testing response in line with the challenge that particular countries were facing. This measure proved to offer very important insights into the data, and to be a key factor.

Finally, a date for the cut-off of the data was needed. The date taken here was 15 July 2020, by which time countries had time to put in place their initial response to the pandemic (especially in terms of testing), and it was becoming clear which had responded better (in terms of mortality) than others. Other dates were equally valid – especially until September, when cases numbers began to pick up again for many of the countries in the dataset and a 'second wave' began. The result of that second wave is beyond this chapter because of the timing of its writing. However, 15 July does seem to provide a reasonable cut-off for most of the countries here in terms of categorising their COVID-19 testing response and in assessing their first-wave COVID-19 mortality.

Once all these factors were put together for OECD countries – so a wider sample of countries than the rest of the book – 25 nations were left. The 'raw' data for the chapter is presented in Table 5.1, with the causal factors (from left to right) being OBESITY (OECD obesity rate), INTARPOP (international arrivals per population), ELD (OECD proportion of people 65+), GINI (OECD income GINI coefficient), COVIDTEST (total COVID-19 tests per thousand people), COVIDM (COVID-19 mortality rate per 1m people), and COVIDCASE (total COVID-19 cases per 1m people).

Among the 25 countries are 10 of those in the rest of the book – France is missing because of its lack of reporting of COVID-19 testing. All testing figures were initially taken from the COVID-19 data section at www.ourworldindata.com and then cross-referenced against national sources to check validity. The figures for GINI vary slightly with the rest of the book simply because these numbers are the most recent available, whereas those in the rest of the book are those from 2017, which is the publication date of the Commonwealth Fund data.

These data were calibrated in the same way as for the rest of the book, with each dataset being graphed and cluster analysis being applied to find crossover points, and the 'calibrate' function in the QCA package in R being applied to generate the fuzzy-set scores.

Results

Low COVID-19 mortality

In the calculation of necessary conditions for low COVID-19 mortality, the combination of TESTCASE+~GINI had a consistency of 0.86 and a relevance of 0.72, and TESTCASE+~OBESITY a consistency of 0.8

Table 5.1: COVID-19 contextual factors and testing for 25 OECD countries

CASE	COUNTRY	OBESITY	INTARPOP	ELD	GINI	COVIDTEST	COVIDM	COVIDCASE
1	AUS	30.40	0.36	0.16	0.33	118.49	4.24	402.00
2	AUT	21.90	3.47	0.19	0.28	77.79	78.72	2116.27
3	BEL	24.50	0.79	0.19	0.26	90.82	844.46	5417.00
4	CAN	31.30	0.56	0.17	0.31	85.13	233.11	2874.11
5	CZE	28.50	0.99	0.20	0.25	55.90	33.15	1245.78
6	DEN	21.30	2.19	0.19	0.26	211.01	105.31	2254.93
7	FIN	24.90	0.58	0.22	0.27	50.33	59.38	1317.70
8	GER	25.70	0.47	0.21	0.29	76.10	108.27	2383.82
9	GRE	27.40	2.81	0.22	0.32	36.69	18.52	372.54
10	ICE	23.10	6.49	0.14	0.26	198.66	29.30	5582.42
11	IRE	26.90	2.21	0.14	0.30	104.69	353.60	5198.68
12	ISR	26.70	0.46	0.12	0.35	127.87	42.86	4893.98
13	ITA	22.90	1.02	0.23	0.33	98.62	578.61	4024.75
14	JPN	4.40	0.25	0.28	0.34	4.44	7.78	177.96
15	KOR	4.90	0.30	0.14	0.36	27.04	5.64	264.31
16	LUX	24.20	1.64	0.14	0.33	449.59	177.32	7917.24
17	NLD	23.10	1.08	0.19	0.29	39.80	357.63	2981.70
18	NZ	32.00	0.75	0.15	0.33	89.10	4.56	248.22
19	NOR	25.00	1.06	0.17	0.26	66.42	46.67	1657.18
20	PRT	23.20	1.58	0.22	0.32	127.45	163.58	4614.33
21	ESP	27.10	1.76	0.19	0.33	82.34	607.62	5488.61
22	SWE	22.10	0.72	0.20	0.28	59.41	549.05	7525.40
23	SWI	21.20	1.21	0.18	0.30	79.12	194.93	3805.02
24	UK	29.50	0.54	0.18	0.36	105.89	662.40	4292.09
25	US	37.30	0.24	0.16	0.39	121.70	412.28	10367.21

and a relevance of 0.77. This means that a combination of TESTCASE (membership of a country in the high tests per COVID-19 case set) or (in Boolean algebra '+' indicates a logical OR) a low GINI coefficient (~indicates negative or low set membership) is a necessary condition. The same logic applies to TESTCASE+~OBESITY.

The truth table (Table 5.2) was then derived with a consistency threshold of 0.8, but which would be identical up to 0.848 or down to 0.775. In addition, a PRI consistency of 0.5 was applied to exclude

Table 5.2: Truth table for low COVID-19 mortality

OBESITY	ELD	TESTCASE	INTARPOP	GINI	OUT	Consistency	PRI	Cases
0	0	1	0	1	1	0.901	0.753	KOR
0	0	1	1	0	1	0.927	0.811	ICE
0	0	1	1	1	0	0.872	0.345	LUX
0	1	0	0	0	0	0.690	0.418	BEL, SWE
0	1	0	0	1	0	0.726	0.393	JPN
0	1	0	1	0	0	0.742	0.477	NLD, SWI
0	1	0	1	1	0	0.687	0.177	ITA, PRT
0	1	1	1	0	1	0.904	0.799	AUT, DEN
1	0	0	0	1	0	0.694	0.278	ISR, US
1	0	0	1	0	0	0.776	0.478	IRE
1	0	1	0	1	1	0.898	0.778	AUS, NZ
1	1	0	0	0	0	0.744	0.499	GER
1	1	0	0	1	0	0.597	0.069	CAN, UK
1	1	0	1	1	0	0.651	0.151	ESP
1	1	1	0	0	1	0.901	0.786	CZE, FIN
1	1	1	1	0	1	0.900	0.780	NOR
1	1	1	1	1	1	0.849	0.591	GRE

a row where a simultaneous subset relation appeared possible – in the third row (Luxembourg).

Directional expectations for the sufficient solution were then assessed, and a decision made to generate the intermediate solution with expectations of a low elderly population, a low GINI coefficient and low international arrivals. These three factors are supported by clinical research suggesting that elderly people are especially susceptible to mortality from the virus, links in research to increased mortality being linked to social deprivation, and international arrivals providing a proxy measure of the degree of cross-border population flows at the beginning of the virus, which is clearly a crucial factor in the spread of a virus in a pandemic. That combination resulted in the following sufficient solution:

Solution term	Consistency	PRI	Coverage	Unique coverage	Cases
TESTCASE* ~INTARPOP	0.913	0.853	0.510	0.141	AUS, CZE, FIN, KOR, NZ
TESTCASE* ~GINI	0.936	0.883	0.478	0.007	AUT, CZE, DEN, FIN, NOR, ICE
OBESITY*ELD *TESTCASE	0.885	0.786	0.376	0.024	CZE, FIN, GRE, NOR
Solution consistency 0.93, coverage 0.65					

The sufficient solution for low COVID-19 mortality has three pathways.

The first pathway has the largest unique coverage and covers five cases, combining high testing per case and low international arrivals. The second pathway covers six cases and combines high testing per case with low GINI. The third pathway combines high testing per case with both high obesity and high elderly population, and covers four cases. All three pathways include the TESTCASE necessary condition.

In these solutions there are no cases deviant for consistency, so that all three combinations of causal factors always lead to low COVID-19 mortality. However, there are three countries which are deviant for coverage – they have low COVID-19 mortality, but do not appear in these solution pathways – Germany, Israel and Japan. The discussion section, in line with other chapters, will explore these deviant cases and the possible reasons for their non-fit with solution terms.

In addition to considering low COVID-19 mortality, COVID-19 cases (per 1m population) were also used as an outcome measure. This created a risk in terms of including both TESTCASE (as a causal factor) and COVIDCASE (as an outcome measure) and so introducing substantial crossover between a causal factor and an outcome measure, but the two had an r of 0.04 only for the uncalibrated data, and 0.10 for the calibrated data, suggesting there is little relationship between the two final measures.

Low COVID-19 cases

For low COVID-19 cases, necessary conditions were TESTCASE+~INTARPOP (consistency 0.91, relevance 0.63) and TESTCASE+~OBESITY(consistency 0.88, relevance 0.76).

The truth table was produced with a consistency of 0.8, but with the same result occurring up to 0.811, or down to 0.778. In addition, a PRI consistency threshold of 0.5 was set. To save space, the truth table is not reproduced here.

The sufficient solution was produced with directional expectations of low obesity, low elderly population, low income inequality and low international travel, given that all these factors appear to be associated with the spread of the virus. However, the same solution is produced with several combinations of the same factors. It was as follows:

Solution term	Consistency	PRI	Coverage	Unique coverage	Cases
TESTCASE*ELD	0.976	0.945	0.521	0.033	AUT, CZE, DEN, FIN, GRE, NOR
TESTCASE*GINI *~INTARPOP	0.917	0.813	0.442	0.082	AUS, KOR, NZ
~OBESITY*GINI *~INTARPOP	0.837	0.628	0.427	0.065	JPN, KOR
~OBESITY*ELD*~GINI *INTARPOP	0.889	0.689	0.421	0.018	AUT, SWI, DEN, NLD
OBESITY*ELD*~GINI *~INTARPOP	0.880	0.674	0.414	0.008	CZE, FIN, GER
Solution consistency 0.864, coverage 0.823					

The solution for low COVID-19 cases therefore has five solution pathways, but with considerable overlap between them – coverage levels for each pathway are high, but unique coverage for each pathway is low.

The first pathway, which covers the most cases among the pathways, combines high tests per case with a high proportion of elderly people. The second pathway has high tests per case in common with the first pathway, but instead of high elderly proportion has a high GINI coefficient and low international travel.

The third and fourth pathways have low obesity in common, combining it with either high income inequality and low international travel, or high elderly proportion, low income inequality and high international travel. The fourth pathway has one case which is deviant for consistency (SWI), in that it has the configuration in that pathway, but has high COVID-19 cases rather than low.

The fifth pathway combines high obesity with high elderly population, low income inequality and low international travel.

Finally, there is one case which achieves low COVID-19 cases, but is missing from the solution – (CAN), and it is therefore deviant for coverage. However, it is important to stress that, given the simplifications of a five-factor model, because of possible measurement errors in tracking the COVID-19 situation, and because complex social factors are not determinant, having so few cases for consistency and coverage suggests that the solutions are robust.

COVID-19 mortality or COVID-19 cases

Finally, the cases were explored in relation to the set of countries with a low solution which fell into the solution set of COVID-19 mortality OR CASES, which means the outcome takes the highest value from either set. This has the effect of requiring cases in the high set to have either high COVID-19 mortality or high case numbers (or both), whereas those in the low set must have both low COVID-19 mortality and low case numbers. As such, using the fuzzy OR method is the most demanding method of joining the two outcomes, requiring countries to achieve low scores in both mortality and case outcomes.

The low set of COVID-19 mortality OR COVID-19 cases therefore comprises the most successful countries in terms of both outcome factors. For this outcome, TESTCASE+~GINI (consistency 0.90, relevance 0.64) and TESTCASE+~OBESITY (consistency 0.88, relevance 0.70) were both statistically and substantively important, and so were regarded as necessary conditions. The truth table was produced with a consistency threshold of 0.788, so slightly below the benchmark 0.8, but lowered to include Australia, New Zealand and South Korea in the solution term, all of which have a PRI score above 0.5, and as such were in the low outcome set. Reducing the consistency threshold slightly, then, increased the coverage of the sufficient solution, while not introducing any deviant cases for consistency. The sufficient solution was produced with directional expectations of low obesity, low elderly proportion, low GINI and low international travel, in line with previous solutions and existing research, and was as follows:

Solution	Consistency	PRI	Coverage	Unique coverage	Cases
TESTCASE *ELD	0.875	0.766	0.522	0.131	AUT, CZE, DEN, FIN, GER, NOR
TESTCASE*~INTARPOP	0.848	0.744	0.586	0.195	AUS, CZE, FIN, KOR, NZ

Solution consistency 0.872, Coverage 0.718

The first solution pathway combines high testing per case and a high elderly population, and the second pathway high testing per case and low international travel. Both pathways have high coverage, but with the second having slightly lower unique coverage.

There are no cases deviant for consistency in this solution term, but two cases deviant for coverage (Germany and Japan).

Discussion of results

The sufficient solution for high COVID-19 mortality as an outcome has three pathways, all of which have high testing per COVID-19 case in common, being combined with low international travel, low income inequality, or high obesity and high elderly proportion. The common factor, however, was high tests per COVID-19 case, emphasising the importance of this factor in achieving low COVID-19 mortality and confirming its key role as a necessary condition.

For low COVID cases, there are five pathways in the sufficient solution. The first pathways two have high tests per case as an important factor, putting test per case at the root of two solution pathways and covering nine countries when combined with either a high elderly population or high income inequality and low international travel. The next two solution pathways have low obesity in common, combining it with either high income inequality and low international travel, or low income inequality and high international travel. The last solution pathway has both low income inequality and low international travel, combined with high obesity and high elderly population.

As such, there are more pathways and more complex solutions for low COVID-19 cases than for low COVID-19 mortality, suggesting that there are more routes to achieving low COVID-19 cases than for achieving low COVID-19 mortality, but also that some of the routes to low COVID-19 cases may not subsequently lead to low mortality as well. It is therefore crucial to try and find the solutions that achieve both outcomes.

The low COVID-19 mortality OR COVID-19 sufficient solution has two pathways only. The first combines high tests per case with a high elderly population (in common with the first pathway of the low cases solution), and the second high tests per case combined with low international travel (in common with the first solution pathway for low COVID-19 mortality). As such, these appear to be the solutions for the countries achieving the best first-wave responses to the virus, and with the first pathway demonstrating that a strong testing regime, even where a large elderly population exists, produces a strong response, and the second that a robust testing regime works well alongside low international travel. As such, the first combination shows testing coping with a potentially higher-risk situation – a high number of elderly people – and the second pathway showing testing working with a factor that should support lower virus transmission – low international travel.

Considering deviant cases gives us additional insight into COVID-19 cases and mortality and how they have played out where the causal factors have not led to the outcomes which the solutions presented earlier suggest. In the low COVID-19 mortality solution these are Germany, Israel and Japan, all of which are deviant for coverage – and so they have achieved low COVID-19 mortality, but not through the same route as the QCA solution.

Despite its internationally lauded testing regime, Germany falls just within the low TESTCAL range of countries, and perhaps suggests that its highly developed track and trace system allowed its testing to be more focused than in other countries (Desson et al, 2020).

Exploring the international COVID-19 tracker data[2] as well as international media coverage, Israel represents a very unusual mix, with a low COVID-19 mortality but a relatively high number of COVID-19 cases, but with a spike in cases at the end of the data period linked to a reopening of the economy, putting it as one of the first countries in that situation (Schulman, 2020). Israel then appears to be one of the first countries to enter a second 'wave' of the pandemic, but sadly other countries which subsequently experienced a similar pattern of infection did not regard what happened there as a warning.

Finally, Japan is unusual in that it did not impose a lockdown until April – well after many other countries included here, but may have had advantages in terms of social factors such as more routine wearing of masks and more socially distant customs such as bowing (rather than handshaking or kissing). Although Japan imposed its lockdown late, it was quicker than many western nations in banning mass gatherings, and this may have also prevented large-scale transmission. Japan looks very much more of an obvious outlier case in terms of its first-wave response to COVID-19 (Fukushima, 2020).

For COVID-19 cases there is one case deviant for consistency – Switzerland – and one case deviant for coverage – Canada.

Switzerland was deviant for consistency in terms of having higher cases than its pattern of solution causal factors ~OBESITY*ELD*~GINI*INTARPOP, and which is shares with Austria, Denmark and the Netherlands, might suggest, as the these other countries have achieved low cases, whereas Switzerland's are high.

Switzerland may have struggled because of cross-border transmission resulting from its geography (Desson et al, 2020).

Canada is just calibrated being in the low COVID-19 mortality set, and is also just in the high COVID-19 case set, while at the same time falling just within the low COVIDTEST set. Its position as a deviant case is therefore explicable in these terms – it is a case on the margins, and one that is clearly doing far better than its near-neighbour the US.

Finally, for COVID-19 mortality OR COVID-19 cases, Germany and Japan are deviant for coverage, but have already been discussed earlier.

Conclusion

The conclusion of this chapter outlines the main points from the earlier analysis, putting its results in the context of health systems research more generally.

The TESTCASE factor, or COVID-19 tests per case, has a strong claim to be the most important causal factor for countries responding most strongly to first-wave COVID, being both conceptually important as it shows the importance of the testing regime needing to be in proportion to the number of cases, as well as empirically central to the solutions we generated. TESTCASE appears in all the solution pathways for low COVID-19 mortality, in two of the pathways for low COVID-19 cases, and in both solution pathways for low COVID-19 mortality OR COVID-19 cases.

The addition of international arrivals as a risk factor in the Economist Intelligence Unit (EIU) report appears justified, even though it is not one that has appeared in existing COVID-19 research, as it appears in solution terms throughout this chapter, so is clearly a factor strongly performing countries have in common. International arrivals appear in the first solution pathway for low COVID mortality (as low), as both low and high pathways in relation to COVID-19 cases (and in all but one solution pathway), and in the solution pathway for low COVID-19 mortality OR COVID-19 cases (as low).

Finally, it is worth considering that the countries that did relatively well in terms of their initial COVID-19 responses were not always, or perhaps even often, those with the highest-ranked health systems. In the Commonwealth Fund 2017 ratings, the UK has the best overall score, despite its substantial problems with health outcomes, but falls clearly in the high set for both COVID-19 cases and COVID-19 mortality. In the 2019 Global Competitiveness Report (Schwab, 2019), Spain was ranked highest for healthcare, but has also struggled in its COVID-19 response. Norway appears in the solution for low

COVID-19 mortality OR low COVID-19 cases, as well as in the high-performing sets for much of this book, but other countries (such as Sweden, the Netherlands and Switzerland) do not. Of these nations, Sweden's approach to the pandemic has been especially controversial in its avoidance of the lockdown measures seen in other countries (Pierre, 2020).

As such, there is a significant disconnect between health system performance in 'normal' times, and the first-wave country responses to COVID, and a great deal of the performance in relation to first-wave COVID-19 depended on the ability of national healthcare systems to put in place a substantial testing system. Among the 11 countries considered in greater depth in this book, Germany has risen to this task, aided by its significant science infrastructure, as well, perhaps, by strong state-based government putting in place local solutions (Beaumont and Connolly, 2020). Germany was also prepared to put in place strong border controls to limit international spread of the virus. Australia and New Zealand quickly put in place both strong testing regimes (per case) as well as robust border controls, with extensive quarantine arrangements that meant international visitors were required to isolate themselves for extensive periods upon entering the country, and did extremely well in terms of their first-wave COVID-19 response as a result. If Germany was aided in its COVID-19 response by its robust scientific infrastructure, its policy response in terms of moving quickly on testing and border controls suggests it still found a strong policy response more quickly than the UK or US were able to, then Australia and New Zealand took advantage of their geography to limit the spread of the virus through their robust border controls and quarantine arrangements. Such an approach may not have been possible in much of mainland Europe, but was certainly possible in the UK. That the UK seems to have moved slowly on testing and on border controls, despite strong voices urging it in that direction during the pandemic (Sridhar, 2020), suggests its response has not been as robust as it could have been had it learned more quickly from better-performing countries.

6

Comparing health systems

Introduction

This book has been about comparing health systems, and this chapter is structured around two final comparisons. The first takes factors which were important in terms of causality from the social determinants, funding and expenditure chapters, and sees how they combine for 10 countries (the inclusion of long-term care expenditure means that New Zealand must be omitted). The combinations of these factors are then explored in terms of their necessary and sufficient conditions in relation to health outcomes. The health outcomes measure has been chosen as the best overall benchmark against which health systems should be judged – if they are generating good health outcomes for their populations, then they are probably doing a good job. Other outcome measures can make a strong case for their importance as well, but as the UK demonstrates, strong health equity can also lead to poor health outcomes, and as the US demonstrates, strong care process measures do not necessarily lead to measures in other outcome measures.

Utilising the health outcomes measure also allows a final comparison, in which the sample of countries is expanded to 31 to see how the causal patterns in that wider sample compare to those in the original 10. Including an outcome measure for the 31 countries means finding a replacement for the Commonwealth Fund health outcomes measure, but a key composite of that measure is the OECD 'preventative life years lost' (PYLL) measure, which provides data for a wider range of countries and so allows a wider comparison to be made.

The chapter first outlines and justifies again which causal factors it will include in its analysis. It then performs QCA using those factors and the Commonwealth Fund health outcomes measure for 10 countries to generate necessary and sufficient solutions. Next, the dataset is expanded to 31 countries, with the same causal factors included, but the OECD's preventable years of life lost (PYLL) measure used as the outcome instead, and QCA is carried out again. Finally, the two sets of results are compared to see which causal outcomes seem to most reliably link to strong health outcomes.

Causal factors

The causal factors taken from the previous chapters were as follows. First, from the social determinants chapter, ~GINI*HEALTHEXP was a necessary condition for high health equity and health outcomes, as well as forming two of the three solution terms in the sufficient solution pathway. These two terms are clearly important in explaining health equity and health outcomes, and so are included in the further analysis that follows.

For health funding, ~VOL was a necessary condition and appeared in both of the sufficient solutions. At the same time, however, GOV also appeared in both the sufficient solutions, and has a robust theoretical explanation for being included. As such, both GOV and ~VOL are included in the analysis that follows.

Finally, for health expenditure there is more of a dilemma as the care process outcomes appear very different to those for health outcomes because there were no necessary conditions for high care and high health outcomes and because the sufficient solution for the achievement of both outcomes was so complex while also covering one country only. Given the concerns over the care outcomes measure, and that for high health outcomes there were necessary conditions of ~HEALTHEXP+LONG, but that the second term, LONG, appears in the sufficient solution with the highest coverage and unique coverage, and is coherent in terms of its increasing importance in health funding, it was also included in the analysis here. Although ~HEALTHEXP is half of the necessary condition, the combination of HEALTHEXP*LONG covers the six cases with high health outcomes. As HEALTHEXP was already included in the analysis because of its role in the social determinants chapter, LONG was added to the list of causal factors in the analysis that follows.

This means that a dataset was compiled for 10 countries (New Zealand is excluded because there are no data on LONG) with GINI, HEALTHEXP, VOL, GOV and LONG as causal factors and the Commonwealth Fund health outcomes measure. The next section presents QCA solutions for those factors.

High health outcomes

The calibrated dataset for the causal factors outlined earlier for 10 countries (New Zealand is excluded because of the lack of data on long-term care expenditures) and high health outcomes is shown in Table 6.1.

Table 6.1: Calibrated dataset for high health outcomes and key causal factors for 10 countries

COUNTRY	GOV	HEALTHEXP	GINI	VOL	LONG	HEALTH OUTCOMES
Australia	0.11	0.30	0.68	0.83	0.02	0.95
Canada	0.20	0.33	0.28	0.95	0.42	0.19
France	0.76	0.24	0.11	0.93	0.33	0.76
Germany	0.94	0.83	0.13	0.07	0.35	0.32
Netherlands	0.85	0.76	0.07	0.25	0.93	0.54
Norway	0.95	0.99	0.01	0.03	0.94	0.89
Sweden	0.93	0.81	0.06	0.03	0.94	0.94
Switzerland	0.03	1.00	0.15	0.33	0.64	0.83
UK	0.77	0.08	0.91	0.19	0.59	0.07
US	0.00	1.00	0.99	1.00	0.06	0.04

From Table 6.1, Australia, France, the Netherlands, Norway, Sweden and Switzerland are the countries with high health outcomes, and from previous chapters, there might be an expectation that Australia might have a different route to high health outcomes than the other countries.

The first step is to calculate necessary conditions. There were two which achieved both statistical and substantive fit.

The first necessary condition was ~GINI, which had a consistency of 0.879 and a relevance of 0.655. ~GINI was a central measure in the social determinants chapter, with research cited there making a strong case for it being important in considering it in relation to health outcomes. Of the high health outcomes countries, France, the Netherlands, Norway, Sweden and Switzerland all have ~GINI, with Australia being the exception – and with the book's analysis having emphasised several times Australia's role in the dataset as an exception case, but emphasising the importance of equifinality in analysis.

The second necessary condition was ~HEALTHEXP+LONG and is perhaps less obvious, but has echoes of the solution from the health expenditure chapter, where it was slightly deceptive in that LONG (along with HEALTHEXP – the opposite of the necessary condition) applied to most of the countries within the solution term, but with Australia and France only having ~HEALTHEXP. This combination of factors has a consistency of 0.919 and a relevance of 0.621. The necessary solution term emphasises the crucial role of equifinality, and that countries with lower health expenditure can have a route to high health outcomes – with AUS being the most significant case.

Table 6.2: Truth table for high health outcomes and key causal factors for 10 countries

GOV	HEALTHEXP	VOL	LONG	GINI	OUT	CONSISTENCY	PRI	CASES
0	0	1	0	0	0	0.705	0.401	CAN
0	0	1	0	1	1	0.850	0.748	AUS
0	1	0	1	0	1	0.984	0.961	SWI
0	1	1	0	1	0	0.501	0.199	US
1	0	0	1	1	0	0.471	0.000	UK
1	0	1	0	0	1	0.968	0.925	FRA
1	1	0	0	0	0	0.699	0.148	GER
1	1	0	1	0	1	0.892	0.825	NLD, NOR, SWE

Of the high health outcomes countries, Australia and France have ~HEALTHEXP, but the Netherlands, Norway, Sweden and Switzerland also have HEALTHEXP – the opposite term – combined also with LONG, so having, in terms of these two causal factors, the opposite of that in Australia and France.

The next step is to produce a truth table with these causal factors. Table 6.2 presents a truth table with a consistency of 0.8, but the same table is produced up to 0.849.

The directional expectations included for the solution were ~GINI (from social determinants)*GOV*~VOL (from health funding). Although both HEALTHEXP and LONG have a case for inclusion, their appearance in solutions has been conjunctional (as well as in relation to the necessary condition). The intermediate sufficient solution this generates is:

Solution	Consistency	PRI	Coverage	Unique coverage	Cases
HEALTHEXP*~VOL *LONG*~GINI	0.906	0.854	0.615	0.545	NLD, NOR, SWE, SWI
~GOV*~HEALTHEXP *VOL*GINI	0.850	0.748	0.218	0.104	AUS
GOV*~CURREXP*VOL *~LONG*~GINI	0.968	0.925	0.221	0.103	FRA

Solution consistency 0.898, Solution Coverage 0.869

The most substantively and statistically important pathway here is the first one, which fits entirely with our expectations for four of the five causal factors (with GOV alone missing as a causal factor). This solution covers the Netherlands, Norway, Sweden and Switzerland, and is a combination of high health expenditure, low voluntary health insurance, high long-term expenditure and low income inequality. These four cases cluster around a solution which is directly in line with the expectations from our previous chapters.

However, as we can see, there are two countries which buck these trends to still generate strong health outcomes – Australia and France.

Australia has been something of an exceptional case throughout the book, with its solution combining low overall expenditure, low government expenditure, high voluntary insurance, low long-term expenditure and high income inequality. What is remarkable about this pathway is that all the casual factors it has in common with the first pathway have exactly the opposite sign, and as such, the necessary condition of ~GINI does not appear in Australia's mix of causal factors. Australia truly is an extraordinary case.

France, on the other hand, is a mix of factors which we might have expected, along with those we would not have. France has low healthcare expenditure, inequality and high government expenditure (which did not appear in our first solution pathway, but is a common factor for three of four countries in it). On the other hand, France also has low overall expenditure, high voluntary health insurance and low long-term expenditure. France is therefore a hybrid, and shows a middle path.

It is hard not to see the power and coherence of the first pathway solution, which coalesces with previous chapters and has high consistency, coverage, and unique coverage. However, it is not the only route to high health outcomes, even if it appears to be the one which is most theoretically and empirically supported.

The next section broadens the analysis to 31 countries in order to compare the results with those just presented.

Preventable years of life lost

To consider whether the solutions from the previous section work on a bigger dataset required an outcome measure that covered a wider range of countries than that provided by the Commonwealth Fund.

To achieve this, the OECD PYLL measure was used, a measure that forms a core part of the Commonwealth Fund health outcomes calculation. This allowed a dataset to be compiled for 31 countries,

Table 6.3: Ranks of the 10 CF countries by health outcomes and PYLL

COUNTRY	PYLL	CFOUTCOMES	rankPYLL	rankCF
AUS	3542.5	0.62	4	1
CAN	4164.3	-0.35	8	8
FRA	4066.6	0.23	6	5
GER	4139.0	-0.18	7	7
NLD	3547.3	0.03	5	6
NOR	3198.8	0.42	2	3
SWE	3251.1	0.55	3	2
SWI	2990.3	0.32	1	4
UK	4185.9	-0.63	9	9
US	6584.5	-0.76	10	10

which is all those among OECD members for which a complete dataset could be constructed.

The first step was to check that the PYLL measure was valid for the comparison. To achieve this, first the rankings of the Commonwealth Fund and those for the PYLL measures were compared. That resulted in Table 6.3.

In Table 6.3 the PYLL column gives the raw PYLL data and the CFOUTCOMES column the raw Commonwealth Fund health outcomes score. PYLL is a measure of preventable years of life lost for a country, and so lower numbers are the highest-achieving countries.

The ranks between the two lists are broadly comparable, with Australia and Switzerland changing places for first and fourth, but no other pairing being more than one ranking score apart. The two raw data columns have an r of -0.778, so an r squared of 0.61, an F value of 12.62 and a p value of 0.007, suggesting a strong association between the two data series.

Having established that the two outcomes measures appear to be compatible with one another, the PYLL measure needed to be calibrated in a way which was compatible with the Commonwealth Fund health outcomes measure. To achieve this, a crossover point was taken by considering the position in the expanded dataset of the countries ranked fifth, sixth and seventh in the Commonwealth Fund data, which found France and the Netherlands falling into the set of high health outcomes countries, and Germany falling into the low set. Because France and Germany fell into different rank orders, and because the data were clearly clustered around two groups of countries, a range of 'crossover' thresholds for PYLL values between 3500 and 4500 were explored. The results using a crossover score for 4100 are shown in the calibrations in table 6.4, but with very similar results being produced up to 4500. Going below 4100 changes the results, making them less consistent as well as providing less coverage in the final solution set, suggesting that the 4100 point, as it produces coherent solutions and is robust across the range 4100–4500, is reasonable.

All the causal factors were then calibrated using the same thresholds as for the factors in the 11–country calibration, again to ensure comparability. That resulted in the calibrated dataset in Table 6.4.

There are 31 countries in the dataset, but with the US included twice. As noted earlier in the book, the US, after the ACA, has been through a significant change in funding, and it is now less than clear whether insurance purchased under the state exchanges is 'compulsory' and so should be regarded as falling under the government and compulsory measure, or under voluntary health insurance. To account for this change, and to see if it made a difference in the solutions it generates for the US, it was therefore included in its pre- and post-ACA form. The first inclusion is based on 2016 measures of the US system counting insurance as voluntary, and is consistent with the rest of the book. The second inclusion of the US counts the insurance introduced by the ACA as compulsory, and so results in a significant change to both the GOVCOMP and VOL measures, with the aim of seeing whether this makes a difference to the way the US health system appears in solutions.

There is one small difference in the calibrated LONG scores compared to those in the rest of the book. Those differences come from two sources. First, the earlier analysis was conducted later than that of the social expenditure chapter, and the OECD had made some small changes to their long-term care measures. To achieve a consistent dataset, these changes were incorporated into the 31–country analysis, but in practice, the only significant change was to Canada, for which the OECD reassessment had taken its measure from the low to high set, with set membership moving from 0.42 to 0.52.

High outcomes (low PYLL measures)

There were no necessary conditions which produced both high (around 0.9) consistency and high relevance (around 0.6). The nearest candidate was LONG+GINI, which had a consistency of 0.867 and a relevance of 0.617, but existing theory and research does not support the GINI condition – in fact the opposite. The decision was therefore taken to not include this combination as a necessary condition.

Table 6.4: Calibrated dataset for PYLL and key causal factors for 31 countries (with US included twice)

CASE	COUNTRY	HEALTHEXP	GOV	VOL	GINI	LONG	PYLL
1	AUS	0.30	0.11	0.83	0.68	0.03	0.18
2	AUT	0.66	0.55	0.21	0.07	0.36	0.29
3	BEL	0.38	0.66	0.14	0.02	0.79	0.49
4	CAN	0.33	0.20	0.95	0.28	0.54	0.52
5	CZE	0.00	0.90	0.06	0.01	0.27	0.76
6	DEN	0.65	0.93	0.05	0.01	0.94	0.39
7	EST	0.00	0.58	0.04	0.39	0.06	0.98
8	FIN	0.05	0.48	0.15	0.01	0.57	0.44
9	FRA	0.24	0.76	0.93	0.11	0.37	0.48
10	GER	0.83	0.94	0.07	0.13	0.45	0.52
11	GRE	0.00	0.01	0.20	0.72	0.02	0.55
12	HUN	0.00	0.12	0.06	0.06	0.04	0.99
13	ICE	0.14	0.89	0.03	0.01	0.76	0.07
14	IRE	0.83	0.19	0.94	0.31	0.83	0.23
15	ISR	0.00	0.01	0.96	0.87	0.09	0.11
16	ITA	0.01	0.50	0.05	0.64	0.16	0.07
17	JAP	0.20	0.94	0.07	0.80	0.61	0.06
18	KOR	0.00	0.00	0.24	0.93	0.21	0.15
19	LAT	0.00	0.00	0.05	0.95	0.05	1.00
20	LIT	0.00	0.08	0.04	0.99	0.10	1.00
21	LUX	1.00	0.91	0.21	0.24	0.65	0.07
22	NLD	0.76	0.85	0.24	0.07	0.96	0.19
23	NOR	0.99	0.95	0.03	0.01	0.99	0.08
24	POL	0.00	0.14	0.31	0.07	0.06	0.97
25	PRT	0.00	0.07	0.19	0.69	0.05	0.50
26	SLV	0.00	0.28	0.97	0.00	0.02	0.49
27	ESP	0.01	0.21	0.14	0.82	0.13	0.10
28	SWE	0.81	0.93	0.03	0.06	0.97	0.09
29	SWI	1.00	0.03	0.33	0.15	0.72	0.05
30	UK	0.08	0.77	0.19	0.91	0.55	0.53
31	US	1.00	0.00	1.00	0.99	0.05	0.98
32	US2	1.00	0.88	0.25	0.99	0.05	0.98

The truth table was produced with a consistency of 0.8 but produced the same result up to 0.848. It is not included here for space reasons. Directional expectations make only small difference to the results, but here, for consistency with the results from the previous section, ~GINI*GOV*~VOL were used. The intermediate sufficient solution that resulted was as follows:

Solution	Consistency	PRI	Coverage	Unique coverage	Cases
LONG*~GINI	0.880	0.788	0.570	0.150	3, 4, 6, 8, 13, 14, 21, 22, 23, 28, 29
~HEALTHEXP*VOL *~LONG	0.819	0.551	0.297	0.141	1, 9, 15, 26
GOV*~HEALTHEXP *~VOL*GINI	0.761	0.593	0.163	0.074	16, 17, 30
GOV*HEALHEXP *~VOL*~GINI	0.921	0.864	0.351	0.018	2, 6, 10, 21, 22, 23, 28
Solution consistency 0.828, Coverage 0.811					

The first solution pathway is a combination of high long-term expenditure and low income inequality. It covers Canada, the Netherlands, Norway and Sweden from the Commonwealth Fund countries, however Canada is deviant for consistency. The full set of countries is Belgium, Canada, Denmark, Finland, Iceland, Ireland, Luxembourg, the Netherlands, Norway, Sweden and Switzerland.

The second solution pathway combines low health expenditure with high voluntary health insurance and low long-term expenditure. It covers Australia and France from the Commonwealth Fund countries. The full set of countries is Australia, Israel, France and Slovenia.

The third solution pathway combines high government spending, low health expenditure, low voluntary health insurance and high income inequality. It includes the UK from the Commonwealth Fund countries, but as a case deviant for consistency. The full set of countries is Italy, Japan and the UK.

The fourth solution pathway combines high government spending, high health expenditure, low voluntary health insurance and low income inequality. It includes Germany, the Netherlands, Norway and Sweden from the Commonwealth Fund countries, but with Germany deviant for consistency. The full set of countries is Austria, Denmark, Germany, Luxembourg, the Netherlands, Norway and Sweden.

As such, there are three cases deviant for consistency – Canada, Germany and the UK, but also two cases deviant for coverage, South Korea and Spain. Overall though, the solution here has very high coverage, and high consistency.

The next section compares the 31-country solution to the 11-country solution to explore how robust the 11-country solution is in the light of expanding the sample.

Comparing the 10- and 31-country solutions

The 10-country and 31-country solutions can be summarised and compared as follows:

10-country solution	31-country solution	Cases
HEALTHEXP*~VOL*LONG*~GINI	LONG*~GINI (INC SWI) + GOV*HEALTHEXP*~VOL*~GINI (EXC SWI)	NLD, NOR, SWE, SWI
~GOV*~HEALTHEXP*VOL*GINI	~HEALTHEXP*VOL*~LONG	AUS
GOV*~HEALTHEXP*VOL*~LONG*~GINI	~HEALTHEXP*VOL*~LONG	FRA

This table shows that the highest coverage sufficient solution for 10 countries is reproduced across two solution pathways across 31 countries.

The first 31-country solution is a simple one, LONG★~GINI, and is a superset of the 10-country solution, which adds two more terms, HEALTHEXP★~VOL. The 31-country solution, then, is one that brings in a range of additional countries including Belgium, Denmark, Finland, Iceland, Ireland and Luxembourg. However, this solution also brings in Canada from the original 11 countries as a case deviant for consistency. The solution is therefore more expansive than the 11-country solution, but the cost of that expansiveness is Canada as being deviant for consistency.

The second 31-country solution pathway covers the Netherlands, Norway and Sweden (but not Switzerland) and comprises GOV★HEALTHEXP★~VOL★~GINI. It therefore has HEALTHEXP★~VOL★~GINI in common with the 11-country solution, but the 11-country solution adds LONG to that solution pathway, whereas the 31-country solution adds GOV instead. The consequence of this change in the 31-country solution pathway is that Germany becomes a case deviant for consistency, and Switzerland is excluded from the solution pathway instead. However, it offers additional cases with which comparisons can be made – Austria, Denmark and Luxembourg (in common with the first 31-country pathway).

There are, then, some differences between the 10-country and 31-country solutions, but expanding the sample to 31 countries gives valuable clues as to a possible simplification of the 10-country solution pathway to LONG*~GINI, as well as making clear which terms are in common between the 10- and 31-country solutions as HEALTHEXP*~VOL*~GINI. ~GINI is at the heart of all of these solutions, re-emphasising its importance at the root of the conjunctures solutions here.

The distinction in the 31-country solution between the pathway containing Switzerland and that excluding it also seems helpful. Switzerland has very low GOV and this does have theoretical importance given the centrality of that factor for high equity and high health outcomes. Both HEALTHEXP*~VOL*LONG*~GINI and GOV*HEALTHEXP*~VOL*~GINI are supported by existing research and by previous chapters in this book, but the lack of GOV in the 10-country sufficient solution does present a different perspective on the data, including Switzerland among the other countries, than the second, which excludes it.

The second and third 10-country solution pathways are combined into one 31-solution pathway, ~HEALTHEXP*VOL*~LONG, which is in common across the two 11-country pathways. In the 31-country solution this pathway covers the cases of Australia, but also France, along with Israel and Slovenia, suggesting that, in terms of the causal factors here, valuable comparisons between these health systems can be made.

The second and third solutions in the table ask us to compare the Australian and French health systems. On the surface, this seems a fairly extraordinary comparison as, although they match the solution term ~HEALTHEXP*VOL*~LONG, they do not match on the other aspects here, with Australia combining those terms with ~GOV*GINI, and France with the exact opposite GOV*~GINI.

Australia and France may initially seem like an unusual comparison, but this is not the first time those two countries have ended up being similarly characterised in the book – they also appeared together in relation to the expenditure factors and health outcomes solution in Chapter 4. In the 11-country solution the countries are placed on different solution pathways because of their different GINI coefficients, but that factor is omitted from the 31-country solution.

The final 31-country solution not included in the table is GOV*~HEALTHEXP*~VOL*GINI and covers the cases of Italy,

Japan and the UK, but with the UK deviant for consistency. This solution pathway does not have an equivalent in the 10-country solution as the UK does not appear on it, but it does open up the potential for additional comparative work between those countries – especially perhaps Italy and the UK. In the 31-country dataset, the UK only just falls into the high PYLL countries (with a calibrated score of 0.53), and so it does significantly better on this measure alone than when the fuller range of indicators in the Commonwealth Fund health outcomes measure are taken into account, and in which the UK does very badly in relation to heart attack and stroke treatments, as well as for cancer survival rates.

The 10- and 31-country solutions, then, are not identical but do have a significant amount in common. Expanding the range of countries produces solutions which are broadly compatible in set-theoretical terms, while introducing the potential for further comparative work, especially for Australia, demonstrating that its mix of causal factors is unusual, but not unique.

In terms of the question as to whether the different configuration of GOV and VOL would lead to the US falling into a different solution term, then both US and US2 appear in the high PYLL solution, with no difference in the causal factors between the two. Both US and US2 appear as CURREXP*~LONG*GINI in one pathway in the high PYLL solution set, suggesting that categorising the US in its pre-ACA form in the book is robust, both for the reasons given earlier, but also because it does not affect the way the country is categorised, at least in relation to health outcomes. Should preventable mortality in the US decrease as a result of the ACA, then it is possible that the pre- and post-ACA US health system might come to be categorised differently, but the system has a very long way to go in terms of improving its health outcomes to reach that point.

Conclusion

This chapter brought together factors identified in Chapters two, three and four as being important in solution terms, defined in terms of being either consistently present necessary or sufficient solutions, and considered their relationship to the Commonwealth Fund health outcomes measure for the 10 countries included in the rest of the book, or for the 31 countries for which full factor data could be gathered, in relation to the OECD Preventable Years of Life Lost measure.

The most important sufficient solution for both 10- and 31-country samples have HEALTHEXP*~VOL*~GINI in common, giving a clear idea though about the pattern of factors which seem to be at the heart of achieving strong health outcomes. That these factors are in common for both 10- and 31-country samples shows that the country sample in the rest of the book is also robust. This solution, although it covers by far the biggest range of countries in the solution set, is not the only one. It is possible to achieve strong health outcomes through other routes, with Australia, which has been an exceptional case throughout the book, achieving this (along with a few other countries, including France).

Including both the pre- and post-ACA measures for the US in the 31-country sample allowed a comparison of their appearance, which was in the high PYLL solution. That both instances had the same combination of causal factors indicated that the decision to include the pre-ACA measures in the rest of the book was legitimate. To look more positively, the post-ACA health system in the US has GOV*~VOL*HEALTHEXP – in common with two of the highest-performing countries in the book, Norway and Sweden. However, the US still differs from those two countries in terms of income inequality and provision of long-term care, with the former factor especially appearing important in relation to social determinants.

Finally, moving from 10 countries to 31 opened up the possibilities for further comparisons by the inclusion of other countries with similar or identical sufficient solutions to those in the rest of the book. There is insufficient space here to take up that challenge, but there are some intriguing possibilities for further work as a result.

The final chapter summarises the book's main messages, considers negative solutions for the outcome measures in the book, explores what can be learned for the health systems of the UK and US, and what can be learned from the most persistently complex case in the book – that of Australia.

7

Conclusion

This chapter presents the book's conclusions, including the key findings from each previous chapter. It also presents the solutions for low performance in relation to social determinants, health funding and health expenditure which were not included in previous chapters, to consider what they can add to our findings. It includes a further discussion of the role of the Australian healthcare system, which has been found to be unusual in its patterns of causal factors and outcomes in previous chapters, as well as a consideration of what the US and UK can learn in terms of health system change. It concludes with a discussion of some general lessons that the book offers and, finally, the strengths and limitations of the book as a whole.

Chapter 2 was concerned with the social determinants of health. It found that countries with high health outcomes have ~GINI as a necessary condition, and there are two sufficient solution pathways to that outcome, ~GINI*EDUC, or BEHAV*~GINI*HEALTHEXP, but with the former having higher coverage of countries, which were France, the Netherlands, Norway and Sweden. For high health equity, ~GINI was again a necessary condition, and the solution with by far the largest coverage and unique coverage was ~GINI*HEALTHEXP, which covered Germany, the Netherlands, Norway, Sweden and Switzerland.

For both high health outcomes and high health equity, ~GINI*HEALTHEXP was a necessary condition, with ~GINI*EDUC*HEALTHEXP forming the sufficient condition for the Netherlands, Norway and Sweden, but with Switzerland deviant for coverage, so also having high health outcomes and high health equity, but not forming a part of the solution set.

As such, for high health outcomes and health equity, low income inequality and high health expenditure were necessary conditions, and the root of the dominant sufficient solution. These two causal factors were therefore carried forward to Chapter 6, which explores the relationship between the most important factors, as well as widening the sample of countries to 31.

Chapter 3 was concerned with health funding and found GOV*~VOL to be a necessary condition for high access, with that combination forming the core of the two sufficient solution pathways (GOV*HEALTHEXP*~VOL and GOV*~OOP*~VOL), and the former covering Germany, the Netherlands, Norway and Sweden, and the latter Germany and the Netherlands (in common with the first pathway), along with New Zealand and the UK.

For health efficiency, the necessary conditions were complex, but included GOV as an alternative in each case, and GOV covers four of the six sufficient solution terms. The sufficient solution with the highest unique coverage was GOV*HEALTHEXP*OOP*~VOL, covering Norway and Sweden, but which can be simplified slightly to GOV*HEALTHEXP*~VOL with slightly reduced consistency, and which covers Germany, the Netherlands, Norway and Sweden. However, other solution pathways exist covering New Zealand, the UK, Australia and Canada, so there are multiple routes to high health efficiency.

For both high health access and efficiency, ~VOL is a necessary condition, with GOV*HEALTHEXP*OOP*~VOL or GOV*~HEALTHEXP*~OOP*~VOL as sufficient conditions, and covering Norway and Sweden, or New Zealand and the UK respectively.

For high access and efficiency, then, high government spending and low voluntary health insurance were core to sufficient solutions, but with different solutions for health expenditure and out-of-pocket expenditure in the two pathways. Both low voluntary health insurance and GOV were taken forward to Chapter 6, as both appear in both sufficient solution pathways.

Chapter 4 was concerned with health expenditure, and considered it in relation to the Commonwealth Fund measures of care, and health outcomes (with the latter in common with Chapter 2). However, the care measure had high scores for countries which have performed poorly in other outcomes, suggesting a care–outcomes paradox, where countries with high care scores often do not achieve high health outcomes. For high care, CURREHAB+PREVENT was a necessary condition, and ~HEALTHEXP*~CURREHAB*PREVENT was the sufficient solution with the highest unique coverage covering Canada and the UK, but with Australia and the US also having high scores, but the Netherlands deviant for coverage.

Health outcome scores produced more reliable results, with ~HEALTHEXP+LONG as a necessary condition (and so including a term we would not have anticipated), but with HEALTHEXP*LONG as the sufficient solution with the highest unique coverage, covering the cases of the Netherlands, Norway, Sweden and Switzerland. Within that sufficient solution, and as HEALTHEXP was already carried forward to Chapter 6 as a result of its inclusion in the solution from Chapter 2, LONG was carried forward as the key solution term for Chapter 4.

Chapter 5 was a little unusual in the context of the rest of the book as it used different data, but comparatively explored contextual factors and testing in relation to the first wave of the COVID-19 pandemic. Solutions, as with other chapters, were conjunctional, but the test per case factor proved to be at the heart of solutions for countries which were most successful in dealing with COVID-19 mortality or COVID-19 cases.

Chapter 6 brought together the factors from Chapters 2, 3 and 4, and led to exploring health outcomes in terms of GOV, HEALTHEXP, GINI, VOL AND LONG. With this combination of factors ~GINI (in common with social determinants) or ~HEALTHEXP+LONG (in common with health expenditure) were necessary conditions, and with the highest unique coverage solution being HEALTHEXP*~VOL*LONG*~GINI – very much in line with existing research. This seems to offer the nearest we can as a template for strong health outcomes, and covers the cases of the Netherlands, Norway, Sweden and Switzerland, which consistently score well across Chapters two, three and four.

These same factors, when the sample of countries was expanded to 31, split the highest-coverage 10-country solution into either LONG*~GINI or GOV*HEALTHEXP*~VOL*~GINI, both of which are also supported by existing research and theoretically coherent, suggesting the solutions are robust beyond the 11 countries considered in most of the book.

Expanding the sample to 31 countries allows possible further comparisons with other countries with the same solution terms, as well as providing the opportunity to explore whether using the causal factors for the US pre and post ACA made a difference to that country's classification, and the solution indicated that this was not the case. However, the post-ACA solution did give the US rather more in common with high-scoring countries such as Norway and Sweden, although key differences remained in terms of its GINI coefficient especially.

It is important to regard the causal factors in these solutions not individually, but as part of large conjunctions, taking into account causal complexity, as well as giving us insights into the crucial contexts in which health systems have to work. If Marmot and other social determinants researchers are correct, and the evidence from this book suggests that they generally are, health systems with very high inequality face different challenges to those with much lower levels of inequality, and with rare exceptions, countries with higher degrees of income inequality seem to be struggling to achieve the same levels of health outcomes. However, that is not the whole story – low inequality is a necessary condition for good health outcomes, not a sufficient one, and other factors need to be taken into account as well.

One of the conditions that turns up in the sufficient solutions for access and efficiency, but also divided those solutions, was out-of-pocket payments. For Norway and Sweden, out-of-pocket payments (along with GOV*HEALTHEXP*~VOL) were high, whereas for New Zealand and the UK, out-of-pocket payments (alongside GOV*~HEALTHEXP*~VOL) were low. What seems to be the case here is that Norway and Sweden have found a way of achieving high access and efficiency, while also making use of higher levels of out-of-pocket payments. From the perspective of the UK, this is a valuable lesson – that such payments do not have to be exclusionary, provided systems are in place to ensure they are managed fairly. It is also the case that Australia, which also achieves high access and efficiency, makes comparatively high use of out-of-pocket payments as well. That such payments can be successfully used can be controversial for advocates of public health systems, but there does seem to be evidence that low out-of-pocket funding countries have something to learn – provided that those payments are located in a health system which also has significant government funding for those who cannot pay them, and low levels of voluntary health insurance to ensure that health equity is maintained.

If Norway, Sweden, Switzerland and the Netherlands have the most consistent causal factors leading to high-performing health systems, then Australia is the country which most consistently (outside of equity) achieves high outcomes with a range of causal factors that are not supported by existing research and theory. It is therefore a critical case in that it appears to offer a very different path to a high-performing health system than these other four countries, and a great deal of space has been spent in different chapters attempting to account for its success.

Australia's high health outcomes solutions in Chapter 6 were ~GOV*~HEALTHEXP*VOL*GINI (10 country) or ~HEALTHEXP*VOL*~LONG (31 country), and neither of these appear obvious routes to high health outcomes. Australia's relatively poor performance in terms of health equity may be a function of its low government spending, and this remains the case even when its more generous health support for its indigenous peoples are taken into account.

Australia has a comprehensive public and private health system and yet manages to spend relatively little on healthcare as a whole, when higher levels of expenditure in other countries are consistently more likely to lead to better health system outcomes. Australia makes comparatively high use of voluntary health insurance and has higher levels of income inequality, but still manages to overcome most health gaps for its white populations, even if it clearly still struggles with those experienced by its indigenous peoples. Finally, Australia spends relatively little on long-term care, when most nations with higher levels of expenditure in this area tend to have better health outcomes.

And yet, despite all of these factors, Australia performs well on most outcome measures in this book. Although there is clear evidence of the health system being under strain (Kay, 2017), Australia is hardly unique in this respect. It is the case, though, that Australia tends not to play a strong role in detailed comparative studies of health systems, where cases such as Canada, the US, Germany, Sweden and the UK tend to dominate. The remarkable success of Australia, despite its pattern of causal factors, demands more comparative work on its health system as there is clearly a great deal to learn from its success, which remains hard to explain from the perspective of the comparative framework of this book.

The book has been concerned with sufficient solutions for countries achieving high solutions for health outcomes, health equity, access, efficiency and care. However, it is equally possible to calculate the necessary and sufficient solutions for countries which are in the low sets for each of these outcomes, and such solutions give indications about the patterns of causal factors which are associated with lower levels of achievement. One such low outcome solution was used in Chapter 6 to compare the pre- and post-ACA causal factors for the US to see if they made a difference to the categorisation of the system. More generally, looking at low outcome solutions means that less promising patterns of causal factors can be identified.

Low outcome solutions

This section will explore some of the negative or low set outcome solutions, exploring the solutions especially with the highest coverage of those outcomes.

For social determinants, the sufficient solution for negative health outcomes and negative equity (calculated on the basis that a low score for either outcome puts countries into this set, based on the boolean logical AND conditional) depend on directional expectations to some extent. If directional expectations of GINI*~HEALTHEXP are used, then the highest coverage solution is GINI*EDU*~CURREXP – so has high income inequality, high numbers of people with pre-secondary education only, and low health expenditure, and covers Australia, New Zealand and the UK with a consistency of 0.931, a coverage 0.378 and a unique coverage of 0.238. This solution pathway includes Australia as its health equity falls into the low set. The solution terms are very much what previous theory and research would have indicated would lead to poor equity and outcomes, combining the findings of Marmot (high income inequality and high levels of pre-secondary education), with those from the OECD (low health expenditure and high levels of pre-secondary education).

If the solution is calculated with directional expectations based more on OECD assumptions (~HEALTHEXP*BEHAV*EDUC) then the highest coverage sufficient solution simply becomes ~HEALTHEXP, which has a consistency of 0.929, a coverage of 0.626 and a unique coverage of 0.325, covering the cases of Australia, Canada, France, New Zealand and the UK. This simplifies the solution term, emphasising the importance of health expenditure for health equity and health outcomes.

Moving on to health funding, the sufficient solution for low access and efficiency (again, calculated using the boolean AND), with ~GOV*VOL as a directional expectation, produces a three pathway solution, each with two countries, so is worth exploring further.

Solution	Consistency	PRI	Coverage	Unique coverage	Cases
~GOV*HEALTHEXP	0.888	0.829	0.459	0.259	SWI, US
HEALTHEXP*~OOP	0.900	0.753	0.397	0.180	GER, NLD
~OOP*VOL	0.978	0.964	0.415	0.207	CAN, FRA
Solution consistency 0.886, Coverage 0.862					

For low access and efficiency, then, the first pathway here has the highest unique coverage solution, and is a mix of low government spending and high health spending.

The second pathway is high health spending (in common with the first pathway), but combined with low out-of-pocket expenditure, but Germany in this pathway is deviant for consistency. The third pathway has low out-of-pocket expenditure (in common with the second pathway), but also high voluntary health insurance. As such, high health expenditure appears in conjunctions in two pathways, as does low out-of-pocket expenditure. ~GOV appears in one pathway, and VOL in another. These solutions therefore overlap, but point to the importance of considering equifinality, with three pathways to negative results for access and efficiency. The first pathway covers countries that have high spending, but low funding from government, and suggests that higher government funding might increase access and efficiency – which would be consistent with the high access and efficiency solution.

The second pathway has high expenditure combined with low out-of-pocket funding, but with Germany deviant for consistency. Perhaps both countries (Germany and the Netherlands) might learn from Norway and Sweden in the high access and efficiency solution, with the pattern of GOV*HEALTHEXP*OOP*~VOL having only one causal factor different with high as opposed to low out-of-pocket payment levels As noted earlier, it would seem that with the right mix of other causal factors, high out-of-pocket payments could be a means of achieving higher efficiency without significantly harming access. This, however, is a challenging finding and will be returned to again in the context of UK healthcare in this chapter. The third pathway combines low out-of-pocket expenditure with high voluntary health insurance. Given that ~VOL was a necessary condition for high access and efficiency, the inclusion of this factor in the low solution set is not surprising and creates a degree of symmetry. But here, for Canada and France, both would require changes to at least two causal factors to move to high outcome solutions.

In Chapter 4 the care outcomes measure appeared rather inconsistent with the countries achieving high scores and with other results in the book. As such, looking at the health outcomes measure only, ~HEALTHEXP*~CURREHAB*PREVENT covers Canada and the UK (consistency 0.937, coverage 0.425, unique coverage 0.250) and HEALTHEXP*~LONG*PREVENT has consistency 0.969, coverage 0.447, unique coverage 0.273 and covers Germany and the US. The only common factor between these two solutions is PREVENT, and with ~PREVENT appearing in one of the high health outcome solutions, there seems to be some link between high preventative expenditure and lower health outcome achievement – at least in the current period, with possible benefits set to accrue in the future if that money is spent wisely. Again, though, these solutions point to the importance of equifinality and causal complexity, with low health expenditure being in the solution term for Canada and the UK, but high health expenditure for Germany and the US.

Negative solutions, then, offer some causal patterns which appear to achieve less successful outcomes, but also emphasise the importance of both equifinality and of causal complexity – there is a real need to understand each country in the context of its causal factors, which allows further comparisons with other similar countries to be made.

Learning from high outcome solutions

What can countries not currently achieving high outcomes learn? Who are most like them, and what can they learn from them?

The United States

The USA scores in the low set of outcomes for every factor considered in the book, except for care, and in that chapter significant doubt accumulated about that Commonwealth Fund measure. Given that the US is by far the highest spender on healthcare, what can be done to improve the system, and from whom could the US fruitfully learn?

As noted in Chapter 6, the post–ACA combination of causal factors for the US appears to be more promising in terms of generating stronger health outcomes than those pre ACA. However, the exact classification of the causal factors, especially in relation to health funding, is now difficult because of the health insurance system no longer being compulsory.

In considering possible paths forward, it therefore makes sense to consider the ACA as *not* having introduced compulsory health insurance, in line with the book's analysis. It is possible to achieve good health outcomes with lower levels of government or compulsory health insurance, with Switzerland and Australia achieving this goal. In terms of health funding, Switzerland, in comparison, makes far lower use of voluntary health insurance than the, whereas Australia has far lower health expenditure. Both Switzerland and Australia then, in terms of funding, are only one causal factor different from the US, but this conceals very significant differences in other aspects of the health systems. The US has high income inequality, in common with Australia, but in difference to Switzerland, and low long-term expenditure, again in common with Australia, but different to Switzerland.

As such, the comparative case most relevant to the US would appear to be Australia (see also Kliff, 2019). In terms of the causal factors explored in Chapter 6, the main difference between the two countries is in terms of the US having high health expenditure, and Australia low. It is clear that the US spends far more on healthcare than other countries, and that reducing that expenditure needs to be a priority for government – indeed it has been since the 1970s. However, accounts of the health system in the US point to significant political lobbying, large-scale public advertising campaigns being launched by lobbying groups which benefit from the present system against attempts at reform, and a gridlocked political system (Skocpol, 1997). Australia does have crucial lessons to offer the US, being also a federal system with a range of common causal health system factors in common, but the Australian healthcare system is facing considerable challenges itself, despite its high outcome achievements in the book, and falls short of the achievements of other countries in relation to health equity. Although Australia spends less than the US on healthcare, its Medicare system is far more comprehensive than that of the US (although under increasing strain (Calder et al, 2019)), and its overall private expenditures are far lower. Perhaps these factors combine to offer the US the clearest lesson – that it is possible to have both a thriving public and private health system at far lower cost – but that the public system needs to be far more expansive, and the private system needs to address its cost issues with greater discipline, and more closely serve the needs of the wider population. The US could do worse than to look to Australia for lessons in improving its healthcare system.

The United Kingdom

The UK's health system is almost the opposite of that the US in terms of most of the causal factors explored here and achieves success in terms of health equity, efficiency and access, as well as in terms of the problematic care measure. The UK appeared as a unique case in terms of its social determinants (although arguably closest to Australia and New Zealand), as having the same pattern of funding as New Zealand, and as having a unique pattern of expenditure (although arguably closest to Canada).

The UK health system is often difficult to characterise in comparative health and welfare studies. On the one hand, the UK can be characterised as having a liberal welfare state (Esping-Andersen, 1990), or as having an 'Anglo-American' capitalism (Jessop, 2002) with its comparatively high income inequality and benefits system which is closer to 'flexploitation' than the 'flexicurity' of Scandinavian models (Viebrock and Clasen, 2009). However the NHS itself is almost socialist in its organisation (Klein, 1986), being overwhelmingly publicly funded and publicly provided to an extent which is very much at the extremes of health systems in the developed world.

The main challenge facing the UK is that it manages to achieve strong equity and access but falls so short of other nations in terms of its health outcomes. Given the solutions in Chapter 6, it is hard not to conclude that one problem is likely to be due to it having the combination of high income inequality and a relatively poorly funded health service. Although the NHS provides equal and fair access, it has not received the same levels of resources as comparable health systems in Europe, and with that funding deficit stretching back decades. So while the NHS might provide comprehensive healthcare, it appears to do so with a relatively low budget, and to a public who may be struggling with more complex health conditions due to the health gaps present in the country. That the UK achieves strong health equity and access might be due to the distinctive way the NHS is organised and care within it is delivered, but its health system is relatively underfunded, and because of its social determinants it is likely to be treating sicker people.

As such, the book suggests three lessons for the NHS, two of which are likely to be uncontroversial to many readers, and one that is more challenging.

A first conclusion is that the NHS needs to spend more on healthcare. There is evidence to show that improvements in health outcomes did happen in the early 2000s, as Labour increased health expenditures, but that they stalled in the 2010s as expenditures were reduced again (Greener, 2018). As the UK continues to lag behind other countries in terms of both its health funding and health outcomes, and has a substantial cumulative deficit in spending going back decades, so there is a compelling case for increased health expenditure.

A second conclusion is that the UK's levels of income inequality are a causal factor in its relatively poor health outcomes. This is a wider public policy issue, but one that clearly addresses the health system. It is true that Australia has been able to achieve strong health outcomes with income inequality similar to the UK's, but the overwhelming evidence in the book points to countries with lower levels of income inequality having better health outcomes. It is also hard not to see the link between this recommendation, which might lead to more progressive taxation, and the first recommendation, the need to increase spending on healthcare in the UK.

The third conclusion is more challenging. Increased government spending is not the only way to provide funding for the health system. It is fairly clear that increasing voluntary health insurance is not a good route forward, but that countries such as Norway and Sweden manage to achieve equitable, high access systems while also having higher out-of-pocket payments in place. It might well be the UK's health infrastructure simply could not support an increase in such payments, or that the revenues generated from them would not exceed the costs of doing so. It might also be that Scotland, where charges for prescriptions and eye examinations have been abolished, would not consider such a move. But it is the case that Norway and Sweden show such a possibility exists, and if it could be achieved without damaging health access and equity, then there is potential to increase health funding through this route.

Strengths and weaknesses

As the end of the book nears, it is worth reflecting on its strengths and weaknesses.

In terms of its strengths, the book presents a consistent method for comparing health systems across a range of different perspectives, showing how those factors interrelate to form patterns, as well as then exploring how they form necessary and sufficient conditions in relation to a range of key health outcomes.

As a result of that analysis, the countries which perform successfully most consistently have been identified, as well as the factors that they have most in common. The method used in the book, QCA, allows for equifinality, and so countries that take alternative routes (especially Australia) have also been identified and discussed at length. Those solutions were tested again in Chapter 6 against a larger dataset and found to be consistent with it.

The book's method, QCA, also represents a further strength, and the book demonstrates the usefulness of that approach in exploring comparative health systems. QCA stresses the importance of equifinality and of causal complexity especially. By identifying necessary and sufficient conditions, and how they relate to key health outcomes, the book presents a range of solutions common to high-performing health systems.

In terms of weaknesses, each chapter has explored a different aspect of health systems, but not every topic has been covered. When put alongside the topics present in Blank et al (2018), the most obvious omission is around the health workforce. The original plan for the book included such a chapter, but the urgency of COVID-19 meant that topic was included instead. The trade-off seems appropriate but does leave a gap.

A second weakness is around data limitations. Most of the chapters are based on robust OECD measures, but they are always proxies and do not fully capture the diversity of different groups in those countries. There are also clear data limitations in terms of the chapter on COVID, which are explored extensively there, as well as in relation to the Commonwealth Fund care outcome measure, which appears to be surprisingly unrelated to health outcomes. Again, the potential issues related to the 'care-outcomes' paradox are discussed at length in that chapter.

Finally, the method used in the book comes with a couple of drawbacks. First, it involves some technical knowledge to fully understand the solutions. An attempt was made to help with this in Chapter 2 by giving a full account of the technical terms in the presentation of results there. Second, the method involves making decisions about the calibration of data and the consistency and coverage of solutions. To try and be as transparent as possible, the full details about calibration are included in the book's Appendix, and discussions about consistency and coverage are included for each solution. The key point here is that QCA involves making decisions about data, but by being as transparent as possible about them, this opens the opportunity for others to agree or disagree about the findings, expanding the debate rather than closing it down.

Conclusion

The book's main messages are in the previous sections and are based around patterns of causal factors that appear to work together in the best-performing health systems across social determinants, health funding and health expenditure. In addition to that, Chapter 5 explored the contexts and policy response (in terms of testing) of health systems to COVID-19.

Although health systems occur in a range of different contexts, only some of them appear supportive of good health outcomes, and there is only so much healthcare systems can do to correct for the additional challenges that substantial inequalities bring. Having a health system with a higher degree of government funding can help balance some of the adverse consequences resulting from wider societal inequalities but is not a panacea in itself. This will be especially the case if healthcare as a whole is underfunded, or if healthcare funding makes significant use of voluntary health insurance. It also seems, in general, that higher levels of long-term health expenditures are linked to better health outcomes, which, in the context of ageing populations and increasing incidences of conditions which are non-curable, is entirely consistent with any expectations we might have had about health expenditures. It also seemed that in the first wave of COVID-19 infections, countries which put in place large-scale, robust testing systems had a significant advantage in terms of both cases and mortality compared to those that did not.

All of these factors, however, do not stand alone but in relation to one another. The book's solutions show again and again the importance of understanding that there are different pathways across the full range of outcomes explored here. It is crucial to take causal complexity and equifinality seriously and to think carefully about what these mean for countries that are currently struggling to achieve good outcomes. In exploring the cases of the US and the UK, both of these factors were taken into account to offer ideas on how these health systems could be improved.

It is clear that the challenges facing health systems are not going away. Increasing health expenditures mean that achieving stronger efficiency has to remain a goal, and this will be even more important post pandemic, when we are likely to see tight government finances and searches for spending economies. In such a time, being able to compare health systems with those from other countries, and find out how things can be made better will be especially important. Health is too important to be based on the prejudices of those who happen to be in power, be they of left, right or central political persuasion. By learning from other health systems there is the opportunity to make things better for us all.

Appendix: Method and data

In QCA set–theoretical relations are the central features of the method, so it is worth explaining these first.

A necessary relation exists where, starting with the outcome we are interested in, we find a range of causal factors that consistently also appear. A simple example will make this clear. To get a graduate job (the outcome), it is necessary to first be a graduate (causal factor). Being a graduate is a necessary condition of getting a graduate job.

However, necessary factors, by themselves, do not guarantee a specific outcome will occur (unless there are also sufficient – which we will explore in a moment). This is because whereas it is necessary to be a graduate to get a graduate job, it is not enough by itself. There are a host of other things that a graduate will probably also have to do – apply for the job, go through a selection and interview process, and so on. So necessary conditions tell us about factors that have to be present (they are 'necessary') to lead to an outcome, but they usually are not enough (sufficient) – by themselves, to achieve that outcome as other factors have to be present as well.

A sufficient relation exists where, whenever we have the cause (or combination of causes), then we also get an outcome we are interested in. It is 'sufficient' to know that, when these causal factors are present, we will also get the outcome. However, just because a cause is sufficient, it does not mean that it is the only way of achieving the outcome. We may have several sufficient solutions (which we will call 'pathways' to an outcome). This is because our causal factors (and others) can be combined in different ways to achieve a specific solution. This approach of having multiple pathways to a solution, rather than a single solution, is called equifinality.

The logic of a sufficient condition is therefore, at least in some respects, the opposite of that of a necessary condition. For a necessary relation we start with the outcome (a graduate job) and then look for consistently present causal factors (being a graduate). With a sufficient relation we consider the other factors that might have to be present and then look for the outcome. So we might say it is sufficient to get a graduate job to be a graduate (a necessary condition), but that might be combined with successfully going through a graduate recruitment programme, or by successfully applying for a specific graduate job, or going through a selection process and passing an interview (among other things), and only when all of these causal factors are in place do we get the outcome – a graduate job. However, there may also be different routes in addition to these (such as having a parent already working in the company).

Now of course, things in the real world are not as simple as this. We are dealing with complex social science relationships, there will always be measurement errors, and no matter how much we like to pretend otherwise, people do not always do as we expect them to. We therefore need to have some means of assessing the strength of both necessary and sufficient relations.

Consistency

Both consistency and coverage can be used to assess necessary or sufficient relations. When considering necessary relations, consistency explores the extent to which instances of an outcome agree in displaying the causal condition (or combination of conditions) which is being assessed for being necessary, while coverage is considered in terms of the relevance of the necessary condition (expressed in terms of how much of the outcome is explained by the conditions). These measures are important, but arguably even more important is their use when calculating sufficient conditions, so most of the explanation here will focus on those.

In calculation of sufficiency, consistency measures the extent to which cases sharing a particular combination of conditions also display an outcome as well. Consistency therefore measures the extent to which a perfect subset relation between the two exists. When we are putting together patterns of causal factors and the particular outcome we are considering, we specify an initial threshold below which we do not consider patterns of causal factors as being relevant in calculating our solutions. This threshold is typically set at 0.8 (out of 1.0) in line with practice in the QCA community, but as we will see, that threshold can be adjusted if doing so can better help achieve a balance between the patterns of causal factors we are considering, and the number of outcome cases that they can help explain.

Coverage

Coverage assesses the degree to which a causal combination (or individual cause in some cases) 'accounts for' instances of an outcome, and so is a measure of the empirical importance of the causal combination we are considering.

Because QCA takes the idea of equifinality seriously, it is possible to have more than one combination of causal factors that are in a sufficient relation with an outcome. In those circumstances, the causal factors can 'overlap' – the same factor or factors can appear in more than one solution. In these circumstances, we need to work out how much of the coverage – the extent to which a set of causal factors is due to each combination of causes. Here, we work out the coverage score for both combinations of factors, as well as when the factors are combined, and so work out the extent to which the solutions are 'unique' or overlap – we effectively apportion the coverage between the different causal pathways. The measure of unique coverage is assesses the extent to which a pattern of causal factors overlaps with the solution on their own, or whether it overlaps with another solution.

In addition to consistency and coverage measures, I also report the 'PRI' measure (proportional reduction in inconsistency) and provides a numerical measure of (roughly speaking) how much it helps to know that a given X is specifically a subset of Y and not a subset of ~Y (Schneider and Wagemann, 2012). The PRI measure attempts to deal with the circumstance where a causal factor (or pattern of causal factors) is a member of both the outcome and the negation of the outcome. This is helpful because it would be illogical for a causal factor (or combination of them) to be in a set-theoretical relation with both an outcome and its negation, and so this measure give us an indication whether this is happening. Generally speaking, when the PRI score falls to a low value (with Schneider and Wagemann providing an example of a low value around 0.35) we should pay careful attention to whether the negation of the outcome, with the same combination of causal factors, produces a higher value.

In all then, when we are calculating QCA solutions, we are looking to balance the consistency of the solutions (from an initial setting of 0.8) with the coverage of those cases. We can generate highly consistent solutions by increasing the threshold higher than 0.8, but this will tend to mean fewer cases will be included in the calculation of our solution. This will lead to cases which are 'deviant for coverage', or not a part of our solution term as we have not managed to include them with the current consistency setting. Equally, we can lower the consistency threshold to cover more cases, but at the risk of creating solutions which create what I will call 'deviant for consistency' cases – cases which have particular causal patterns which our consistency threshold suggests should have a particular outcome, but in fact do not.

As such, to put all these terms together, in QCA we are generally looking for combinations of causal conditions which have a high degree of consistency (0.8 to start with) in relation to an outcome. When we find such conditions, we are interested in how important they are, and coverage (and unique coverage) gives us an indication of this – with coverage measuring the extent of the outcome that the causal combination 'covers'. Coverage has a theoretical maximum of 1.0 where the causal combinations would completely cover the outcome, but in reality it is extremely unlikely coverage scores come any near this idea.

Calibration

Calibration of the data, as noted earlier, was derived using the direct method, with the key 'crossover' point (the 0.5 value, which in fuzzy-set analysis is the point of indeterminacy, where a value can be said to be neither in nor out of the set) derived through an interactive process. First, I graphed the data to look for a clear 'gap' or 'break', comparing that crossover to what we know about countries from existing research (for example, the UK is known, internationally, to be a relatively slow spender on healthcare, and the US a high spender). I then performed cluster analysis on the data to try and identify the crossover, as well as the 'low' and 'high' thresholds of the data, comparing those results to those derived from graphing. Finally, the data were calibrated using the 'calibrate' command in the QCA package in R (Dusa, 2018).

The results of data calibration are perhaps most easily explained through the use of graphs. On each X axis I have the 'raw' data, and on the Y axis the calibrated scores. All data in the project are shown in the figures, along with commentaries where results are at all complex or contentious.

For health expenditure, the US is a clear outlier (at the top right of the graph) and New Zealand (bottom left) clearly the lowest spenders. However, in deriving 'high' spenders, the top three spenders (US, Switzerland and Norway) are unequivocally 'high' spenders and so are at or close to the 1.0 threshold. Below that we have three countries (Germany, the Netherlands and Sweden) which are clearly high spenders as well, and which so fall around 0.8 in the set of health expenditure. We then have three spenders below $5000, which acts as the 'crossover' point. At the bottom end, a spend of $4000 was treated as the 'low' value, with New Zealand falling slightly below that. At the top end, I treated $6000 as the threshold for high spending as eight of the 11 countries were below this point, and this emphasised that countries spending above this level were very much exceptions.

There is a clear gap in the data here between low and high pre-secondary education sets, making the data a little more challenging

Figure A1: Health expenditure calibration

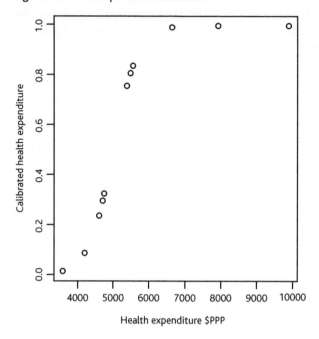

Figure A2: Behavioural factors calibration

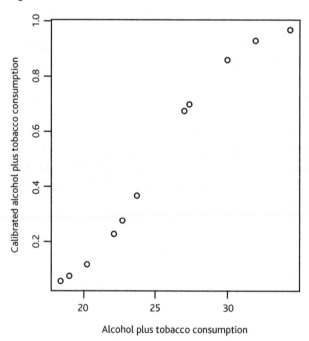

Figure A3: GINI coefficient calibration

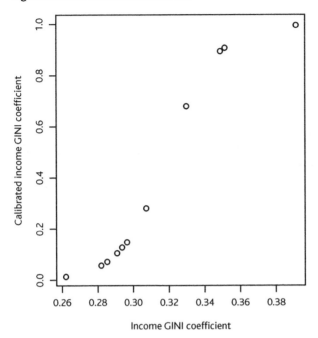

Figure A4: Pre-secondary education calibration

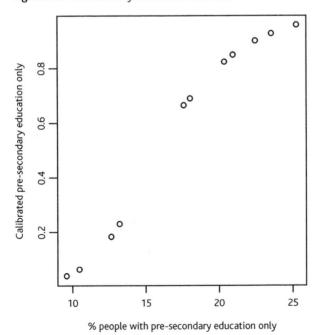

to interpret because of the 4 countries clustered at the low end of the chart and finding a balanced calibration.

There is a clear outlier in low government funding set (the US), but a gap between low and high at 75 per cent funding. However this does mean that there are only four countries in the low government funding set.

The voluntary health insurance calibration is one of the more difficult here. This is because of the cluster of cases in the 5–10 per cent range, which could reasonably be included in either the high or low set. Here I took the decision to put the crossover point at 10 per cent, as this corresponded with the cluster analysis and was defendable. However, I also ran all the analysis in the following pages taking a figure of 7 per cent instead, which put more cases into the 'high' set. The difference from the results that follow was marginal, not changing the substantive results but with New Zealand moving to being a case deviant for consistency in the results including this factor. As such, I kept the calibration as I have described to as it achieved a better balance between solution consistency and coverage for the cases.

The out-of-pocket calibration again has a significant outlier at the top end, but if that value is removed, the crossover point at US$ 740 becomes more obvious, as well as the gap between the high and lower out-of-pocket spenders becoming clearer than is immediately obvious on Figure A7.

There is clearly a cluster of lower spenders on curative and rehabilitative expenditure, so that only three countries fall in the 'high' set.

For long-term care the two very low levels make the crossover point (17.5 per cent) less obvious, but once the data are replotted and cluster analysis recalculated without them, it becomes clearer that this represents a valid gap in the data.

Preventative care presents us with a challenge in that the three data points in the middle of the figure could fall either above or below the crossover point. The choice this presents is to remove the three data points in the middle (reducing the dataset to seven cases), or to make a decision to put the crossover to the left of the cluster (so having only three 'low' cases) or to the right, so having only three 'high' cases). As the full range of data runs from under 2 per cent up to 5 per cent, putting the threshold for 'high' at around 4 per cent, as would be needed to put the cluster into the lower set, would seem to be at least empirically less sound. Given that we do not have benchmarks or strong theory, I therefore used 3.5, which is broadly the middle value of the data, as the crossover point, which is also more demanding of

Figure A5: Government health funding calibration

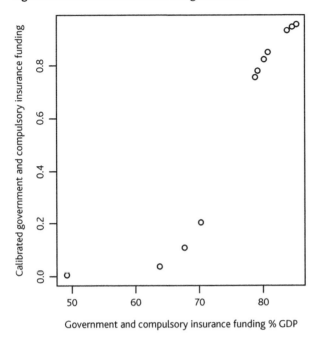

Government and compulsory insurance funding % GDP

Figure A6: Voluntary health insurance calibration

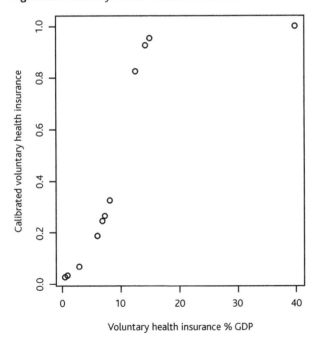

Voluntary health insurance % GDP

Figure A7: Out-of-pocket funding calibration

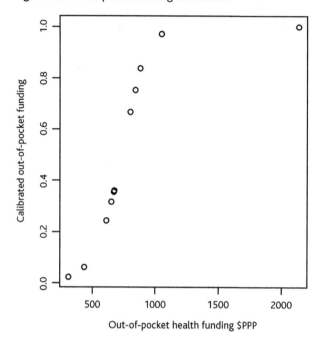

Figure A8: Curative and rehabilitative expenditure calibration

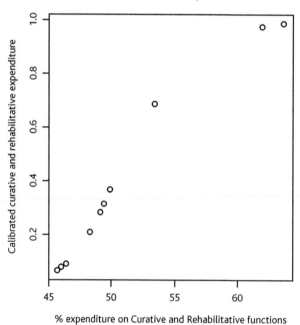

Figure A9: Long-term care expenditure calibration

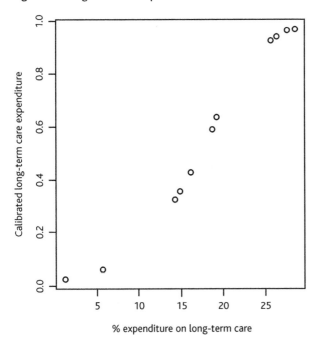

Figure A10: Preventative care expenditure calibration

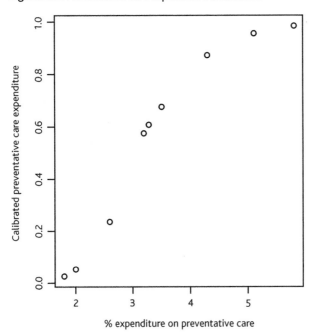

the data as a causal factor as it makes calibrated scores higher, and so the requirement for sufficient subset solutions are more challenging.

The calibration of the Commonwealth Fund outcome scores presents a dilemma. The outcome scores are index constructs, or scores which have been combined from a number of sources, then subject to standardisation, and then averaged. As such, the scores above zero are not objectively 'high' and the scores below zero are not objectively 'low', in the sense that they are not compared to an external standard which is the ideal for calibrating outcome measures (Ragin, 2008, 2014).

Instead, the Commonwealth Fund outcome measures are scores which are explicitly produced through comparison with other countries in the sample. As I have demonstrated in the Introduction, the sample of countries, although not entirely representative of developed countries, does have credibility in including countries from a range of welfare and health typologies, and so can claim a degree of representativeness. It is also the case that, although the scores are standardised and averaged against one another, they are meant to be used in ranking countries (and are used as such by policymakers (Greener, 2016)), and the scores, in relation to the zero measure, are meant to represent countries that are performing well or poorly.

As such, when calibrating the Commonwealth Fund scores, zero was used as a crossover point in all the calibrations of measures. This seemed to be both a consistent and justifiable position. The use of the zero crossover does not change the ranking of countries, but does mean that marginal scores (Germany scoring 0.01 for equity, the Netherlands 0.03 for health outcomes) have to be interpreted in that light. But given the lack of objective external measures to compare and benchmark the scores against, this solution, although flawed, seemed like the best compromise.

Notes

Chapter 1

[1] https://www.commonwealthfund.org/international-health-policy-center/countries

Chapter 2

[1] https://www.apha.org/topics-and-issues/health-rankings
[2] https://www.aihw.gov.au/reports/australias-welfare/indigenous-income-and-finance
[3] https://www.tobaccoinaustralia.org.au/chapter-8-aptsi/8-3-prevalence-of-tobacco-use-among-aboriginal-peo
[4] https://www.aihw.gov.au/reports/life-expectancy-death/deaths/contents/life-expectancy
[5] https://www.aihw.gov.au/reports/australias-welfare/indigenous-education-and-skills

Chapter 3

[1] https://www.health.gov.au/health-topics/private-health-insurance/what-private-health-insurance-covers/out-of-pocket-costs

Chapter 5

[1] For example https://www.bsg.ox.ac.uk/research/research-projects/coronavirus-government-response-tracker
[2] https://www.bsg.ox.ac.uk/research/research-projects/coronavirus-government-response-tracker

References

Arrow, K. (1963) 'Uncertainty and the Welfare Economics of Medical Care', *American Economic Review*, 53(5), pp 941–973.

Bambra, C. (2011) *Work, Worklessness, and the Political Economy of Health.* Oxford: Oxford University Press.

Bambra, C. (2017) *Health Divides: Where You Live Can Kill You.* Bristol: Policy Press.

Beaumont, P. and Connolly, K. (2020) 'Covid-19 Track and trace: What can UK learn from countries that got it right?; Pledge of "world-beating" system will have to look to likes of South Korea and Germany', *The Guardian*, 21 May.

Beland, D. and Waddan, A. (2012) *The Politics of Policy Change: Welfare, Medicare and Social Security Reform in the United States.* Washington: Georgetown University Press.

Bevan, G. *et al.* (2014) *The Four Health Systems of the United Kingdom: How Do They Compare?* London: The Health Foundation and Nuffield Trust.

Blank, R. H., Burau, V. and Kuhlmann, E. (2018) *Comparative Health Policy.* London: Palgrave.

Boslaugh, S. (2013) *Healthcare Systems Around the World: A Comparative Guide.* London: Sage.

Calder, R., Dunkin, R., Rochford, C., and Nichols, T. (2019) *Australian Health Services: Too Complex to Navigate.* Melbourne: Mitchell Institute.

Case, A. and Deaton, A. (2020) *Deaths of Despair and the Future of Capitalism.* Princeton, NJ: Princeton University Press.

Davis, K., Stremikis, K., Squires, D., and Schoen, C. (2014) *Mirror, Mirror on the Wall: How the Performance of the U.S. Health Care System Compares Internationally.* New York: Commonwealth Fund.

Deaton, A. (2015) *The Great Escape: Health, Wealth and the Origins of Inequality.* Princeton, NJ: Princeton University Press.

Desson, Z., (2020) 'Europe's Covid-19 Outliers: German, Austrian and Swiss Policy Responses During the Early Stages of the 2020 Pandemic', *Health Policy and Technology*, p S2211883720300964. doi: 10.1016/j.hlpt.2020.09.003.

Dusa, A. (2018) *QCA with R: A Comprehensive Resource.* London: Springer.

Economist Intelligence Unit (2020) *How Well Have OECD Countries Responded to the Coronavirus Crisis?* London: Economist Intelligence Unit.

Esping-Andersen, G. (1990) *The Three Worlds of Welfare Capitalism.* Princeton, NJ: Princeton University Press.

Fukushima, G. (2020) 'Japan's response to COVID-19: A preliminary assessment', *The Japan Times*, 5 May. Available at: https://www.japantimes.co.jp/opinion/2020/05/05/commentary/japan-commentary/japans-response-covid-19-preliminary-assessment/

Giamo, S. (2018) *Reforming Health Care in the United States, Germany, and South Africa.* New York: Palgrave.

Goldacre, B. and OpenSAFELY Collaborative (2020) 'Factors associated with COVID-19-related hospital death in the linked electronic health records of 17 million adult NHS patients', *medRxiv.* Available at: https://doi.org/10.1101/2020.05.06.20092999

Gordon, C. (2009) *Dead on Arrival: The Politics of Health Care in Twentieth Century America.* Princeton, NJ: Princeton University Press.

Greener, I. (2008) 'Expert Patients and Human Agency: Long-term Conditions and Giddens Structuration Theory', *Social Theory and Health*, 6(4), pp 273–290.

Greener, I. (2016) 'An Argument Lost by Both Sides? The Parliamentary Debate over the 2010 NHS White Paper', in Powell, M., Exworthy, M. and Mannion, R. (eds) *Dismantling the NHS? Evaluating the Impact of Health Reforms.* Bristol: Policy Press, pp 105–125.

Greener, I. (2018) 'Learning from New Labour's Approach to the NHS', in Needham, C., Heins, E. and Rees, J. (eds) *Social Policy Review 30.* Bristol: Bristol University Press.

Greener, I. (2020) 'Healthcare Funding and Its Relationship to Equity and Outcomes: A QCA Analysis of Commonwealth Fund and OECD Data', *Journal of European Social Policy*, 30(4), pp 480–494. doi: 10.1177/0958928720905290.

Greenhalgh, T. (2009) 'Patient and Public Involvement in Chronic Illness: Beyond the Expert Patient', *BMJ*, 338 (17 February), p b49.

Haidt, J. (2013) *The Righteous Mind: Why Good People Are Divided by Politics and Religion.* London: Penguin.

Healy, J., Sharman, E. and Lokuge, B. (2006) 'Australia: Health System Review', *Health Systems in Transition (World Health Organization)*, 8(5), pp 1–158.

Hernstein, R. and Murray, C. (1996) *The Bell Curve: Intelligence and Class Structure in American Life.* London: Simon & Schuster.

Illich, I. (1977a) *Disabling Professions.* London: Marion Boyars.

Illich, I. (1977b) *Limits to Medicine.* Harmondsworth: Penguin.

Immergut, E. (1992a) *Health Politics: Interests and Institutions in Western Europe.* New York: Cambridge University Press.

Immergut, E. (1992b) 'The Rules of the Game: The Logic of Health Policy-making in France, Switzerland and Sweden', in Steinmo, S., Thelen, K. and Longstreth, F. (eds) *Structuring Politics: Historical Institutionalism in Comparative Analysis*. Cambridge: Cambridge University Press, pp 57–89.

Jessop, B. (2002) *The Future of the Capitalist State*. Cambridge: Polity.

Johnson, J., Stoskopf, C. and Shi, L. (2017) *Comparative Health Systems*. Burlington, MA: Jones and Bartlett Publishers.

Kay, A. (2017) 'Policy Failures, Policy Learning and Institutional Change: The Case of Australian Health Insurance Policy Change', *Policy & Politics*, 45(1), pp 87–101.

Kenworthy, L. (2019) *Social Democratic Capitalism*. Oxford: Oxford University Press.

Kirby, T. (2020) 'Evidence Mounts on the Disproportionate Effect of COVID-19 on Ethnic Minorities', *The Lancet Respiratory Medicine*, 8(6), pp 547–548. doi: 10.1016/S2213-2600(20)30228-9.

Klein, R. (1986) 'Why Britain's Conservatives Support a Socialist Health Care System', *Health Affairs*, 4(1), pp 41–58.

Kliff, S. (2019) 'What Australia Can Teach America About Health Care', *Vox*, 15 April.

Kotlikoff, L. and Hagist, C. (2005) 'Who's Going Broke? Comparing Growth in Healthcare Costs in Ten OECD Countries', *University of Frieberg Working Paper*, 7.

Lakoff, G. (2016) *Moral Politics: How Liberals and Conservatives Think*. Chicago, IL: University of Chicago Press.

Lawson, N. (1991) *The View from No. 11*. London: Corgi.

Le Fanu, J. (2018) *Too Many Pills: How Too Much Medicine Is Endangering Our Health and What We Can Do About It*. London: Little Brown.

Marmot, M. (2012) *Status Syndrome: How Your Social Standing Directly Affects Your Health*. London: Bloomsbury.

Marmot, M. (2015) *The Health Gap: The Challenge of an Unequal World*. London: Bloomsbury.

Marmot, M. and Wilkinson, R. (2005) *Social Determinants of Health*. Oxford: Oxford University Press.

McCartney, M. (2012) *The Patient Paradox: Why Sexed Up Medicine Is Bad for Your Health*. London: Pinter and Martin Ltd.

Moran, M. (1995) 'Three Faces of the Health Care State', *Journal of Health Politics, Policy and Law*, 20(3), pp 767–782.

Moran, M. (1999) *Governing the Healthcare State: A Comparative Study of the United Kingdom, the United States and Germany*. Manchester: Manchester University Press.

Mullainathan, S. and Shafir, E. (2013) *Scarcity: Why Having So Little Means So Much*. London: Penguin.

Nixon, J. and Ulmann, P. (2006) 'The Relationship Between Health Care Expenditure and Health Outcomes', *European Journal of Health Economics*, 7(7), pp 7–18.

OECD (2017) 'What Has Driven Life Expectancy Gains in Recent Decades? A Cross-country Analysis of OECD Member States', in *Health at a Glance*. Paris: Organisation for Economic Co-operation and Development.

OECD (2019) *Deriving Preliminary Estimates of Primary Care Spending Under the SHA 2011 Framework*. Paris: Organisation for Economic Co-operation and Development.

OECD, Eurostate and World Health Organization (2017) *A System of Health Accounts 2011*. Paris: OECD Publishing.

OECD and European Observation on Health Systems and Policies (2019a) 'Germany: Country Health Profile 2019'. Available at: https://www.oecd-ilibrary.org/content/publication/36e21650-en

OECD and European Observation on Health Systems and Policies (2019b) 'Netherlands: Country Health Profile 2019'. Available at: https://www.oecd-ilibrary.org/content/publication/9ac45ee0-en

O'Mahony, S. (2016) 'Medical Nemesis 40 Years On: The Enduring Legacy of Ivan Illich', *Journal of the Royal College of Physicians of Edinburgh*, 46, pp 134–139.

O'Mahony, S. (2019) *Can Medicine Be Cured? The Corruption of a Profession*. London: Apollo.

Peckham, S. and Exworthy, M. (2003) *Primary Care in the UK: Policy, Organisation and Management*. Basingstoke: Palgrave.

Pierre, J. (2020) 'Nudges Against Pandemics: Sweden's COVID-19 Containment Strategy in Perspective', *Policy and Society*, 39(3), pp 1–16. doi: 10.1080/14494035.2020.1783787.

Ragin, C. (2000) *Fuzzy-Set Social Science*. Chicago, IL: University of Chicago Press.

Ragin, C. (2008) *Redesigning Social Inquiry: Fuzzy Sets and Beyond*. Chicago, IL: University of Chicago Press.

Ragin, C. (2014) *The Comparative Method: Moving Beyond Qualitative and Quantitative Strategies*. Oakland, CA: University of California Press.

Ragin, C. and Fiss, P. (2016) *Intersectional Inequality: Race, Class, Test Scores and Poverty*. Chicago, IL: University of Chicago Press.

Reibling, N., Ariaans, M. and Wendt, C. (2019) 'Worlds of Healthcare: A Healthcare System Typology of OECD Countries', *Health Policy*, 123(7), pp 611–620. doi: 10.1016/j.healthpol.2019.05.001.

Sandel, M. (2020) *The Tyranny of Merit: What's Become of the Common Good?* London: Penguin.

Schneider, C. and Wagemann, C. (2012) *Set-Theoretical Methods for the Social Sciences.* Cambridge: Cambridge University Press.

Schneider, E. (2017) *Mirror Mirror 2017.* New York: Commonwealth Fund.

Schrecker, T. and Bambra, C. (2015) *How Politics Makes Us Sick: Neoliberal Epidemics.* Basingstoke: Palgrave Macmillan.

Schulman, M. (2020) 'Sudden Implosion of Israel's COVID-19 Response Might Prove Netanyahu's Undoing', *Newsweek*, 21 July. Available at: https://www.newsweek.com/netanyahu-covid-response-israel-chaos-1519456

Schwab, K. (2019) *The Global Competitiveness Report 2019.* Geneva: World Economic Forum.

Self, S. and Grabowski, R. (2003) 'How Effective Is Public Health Expenditure in Improving Overall Health? A Cross-country Analysis', *Applied Economics*, 35, pp 835–845.

Skocpol, T. (1997) *Boomerang: Health Care Reform and the Turn Against Government.* London: W.W. Norton and Co.

Sridhar, D. (2020) 'This is what you should be demanding from your government to contain the virus; Four months in, we know what works against coronavirus. These are eight important lessons from east Asia', *The Guardian*, 4 May.

Starr, P. (2013) *Remedy and Reaction: The Peculiar American Struggle Over Health Care Reform.* London: Yale University Press.

Stegenga, J. (2018) *Medical Nihilism.* Oxford: Oxford University Press.

Tuohy, C. (1999) *Accidental Logics: The Dynamics of Change in the Health Arena in the United States, Britain, and Canada.* New York: Oxford University Press.

Tuohy, C. (2018) *Remaking Policy: Scale, Pace and Political Strategy in Health Care Reform.* Toronto: University of Toronto Press.

Viebrock, E. and Clasen, J. (2009) 'Flexicurity and Welfare Reform: A Review', *Socio-Economic Review*, 7(2), pp 305–331.

WHO (2020) 'WHO Director-General's opening remarks at the media briefing on COVID-19 – 16 March 2020'. Available at: https://www.who.int/dg/speeches/detail/who-director-general-s-opening-remarks-at-the-media-briefing-on-covid-19—16-march-2020

Wilkinson, R. and Pickett, K. (2010) *The Spirit Level: Why Equality Is Better for Everyone.* London: Penguin.

Wilkinson, R. and Pickett, K. (2018) *The Inner Level: How More Equal Societies Reduce Stress, Restore Sanity and Improve Everyone's Well-being.* London: Allen Lane.

Wilsford, D. (1994) 'Path Dependency, or Why History Makes It Difficult, but Not Impossible, to Reform Health Care Services in a Big Way', *Journal of Public Policy*, 14, pp 251–283.

Wilsford, D. (1995) 'States Facing Interests: Struggles over Health Care Policy in Advanced Industrial Democracies', *Journal of Health Politics, Policy and Law*, 20, pp 571–613.

World Health Organization (2000) *The World Health Organization Report 2000: Health Systems Improving Performance*. Geneva: World Health Organization.

Index

References to figures appear in *italic* type;
those in **bold** type refer to tables.

A

access to health services
  high 71, 72–75, **72**, **73**, 81–82,
    82–83, 85–86, 141–142
  high efficiency and high 79–81, **79**,
    80, 85, 86, 87, 142, 146
  measure 15–16, **16**
  and risk of moral hazard 63–64, 66
Affordable Care Act (ACA) 2010 9, 66,
    69, 112, 114, 134, 140, 148
alcohol consumption 5, 6, **6**, 31, 33,
    34, 44, 50
  see also behavioural characteristics
American Public Health
    Association 30, 32
Australia 58–61, 144–145
  comparing 10- and 31- country
    solutions 137, 138
  COVID-19 **119**, **120**, 123, 127
  health outcome gaps 50–51, 60
  health outcomes and key causal
    factors 130, **130**, 131, **131**, 132,
    144–145
  high outcomes (low PYLL
    measures) 136
  lessons to offer US for improving
    healthcare system 148–149
  life expectancy *31*, 51, 60
  Medicare 59, 60
  public health 50
  PYLL and key causal factors **135**
  ranking by health outcomes and
    PYLL 133, **133**
Australia, health expenditure **12**, 60,
    99, **99**, **100**
  and care and health outcomes 105,
    105, 106, **106**, 108
  and care score **101**, 102, **102**, 106, 107
  Commonwealth Fund care process
    score **18**
  Commonwealth Fund health
    outcomes score **14**
  and health outcomes 103, **103**, 104,
    104, 108, 109–110
Australia, health funding 9, **9**, 59–60,
    70, **70**
  and access 73, **73**, 74, 75, 82–83, 87
  and access and efficiency 79, **79**, 80,
    80, 85, 87

clustering **71**
Commonwealth Fund access
    measure **16**
Commonwealth Fund efficiency
    score **17**
  and efficiency **75**, 76, 77, **77**, 78, 84,
    85, 86
Australia, social determinants of
    health **6**, **34**, **35**, 50–51, 61
Commonwealth Fund health equity
    measure **15**
Commonwealth Fund health
    outcomes score **14**
  and health equity **43**, **44**
  and health equity and health
    outcomes **46**, **47**, 51
  and health outcomes **38**, 39, **39**, 42,
    50, 54, 146

B

behavioural characteristics 34, 37
  country clustering 35–36, **35**
  and health equity **43**, **43**, 44, **44**
  and health equity and health
    outcomes **46**, **47**
  and health outcomes 34, **38**, **39**,
    40, 42
Blank, R.H. 1–2, 93, 94, 98, 151
Boslaugh, S. 22
Burau, V. 1–2

C

Canada 110–111, 146, 147
  comparing 10- and 31- country
    solutions 137
  COVID-19 **119**, **120**, 126
  health gap 111
  health outcomes and key causal
    factors 130, **131**
  high outcomes (low PYLL
    measures) 136, 137
  life expectancy *31*
  Medicare 110, 111
  PYLL and key causal factors 134, **135**
  ranking by health outcomes and
    PYLL **133**
Canada, health expenditure 12, **12**, 99,
    99, **100**, 111
  and care and health
    outcomes **105**, **106**

and care score 101, **101**, 102, **102**, 106, 107
Commonwealth Fund care process score **18**
Commonwealth Fund health outcomes score **14**
and health outcomes 103, **103**, **104**, 147
Canada, health funding 9, **9**, **70**, 110–111
and access **72**, **73**
and access and efficiency 79, **79**, **80**, 146
clustering 71, **71**
Commonwealth Fund access measure **16**
Commonwealth Fund efficiency score **17**
and efficiency **75**, 76, 77, **77**, 78, 84, 86
Canada, social determinants of health 6, **6**, **34**, **35**, 36, 111
Commonwealth Fund health equity measure **15**
Commonwealth Fund health outcomes score **14**
and health equity **43**, **44**
and health equity and health outcomes **46**, **47**
and health outcomes **38**, 39–40, **39**, 146
'care and outcomes paradox' 94, 108–109
care process measures, Commonwealth Fund 17–18, **18**, 107, 109, 129
care score, health
high 100–102, **101**, **102**, 106–107, 142
high outcomes score and high 105–106, **105**, **106**, 108–109, 142
case studies 22–23
Australia 58–61
Canada 110–111
France 91–92
Germany 54–57
Netherlands 26–28
New Zealand 89–91
Norway 23–24
Sweden 25–26
Switzerland 57–58
UK 87–89
US 112–114
choice of countries for comparison 2–4
Clinton, Bill 66
Commonwealth Fund 3, 9, 22
health expenditure outcomes 17–19, **18**

health funding outcomes 15–17, **16**, **17**
social determinants outcomes 13–15, **14**, **15**
comparing health systems 128–140
causal factors 129
comparing 10- and 31- country solutions 137–139, 139–140, 143
high health outcomes 129–132, **130**, **131**, 143
high health outcomes (low PYLL measures) 134–137
key findings 143–145
methodology 128
preventable years of life lost 132–134, **133**, **135**
selection of countries for comparison 2–4
compulsory health insurance 7–8, 64
see also government and compulsory health insurance funding
co-payments for healthcare 7, 65
France 91
Germany 55
Netherlands 27, 28
Norway 23
Sweden 25, 26
UK 88
COVID-19 12–13, 115–127, 143
COVID-19 mortality or COVID-19 cases 123–124, 124–125, 126
data and calibration 116–118, **119**
health system ranking and success in response to 126–127
international arrivals and 117, 118, **119**, 120, **120**, 121, 122, 123, 125, 126
low COVID-19 cases 121–123, 124, 125–126
low COVID-19 mortality 118–121, **120**, 124, 125
risk factors 115–116
tests per COVID-19 case 117–118, 118–119, **120**, 121, 122, 123, 126, 143
curative and rehabilitative expenditure 10, 11, **12**, 97, 99, **99**, **100**
high care score and high outcomes score **105**, 106, **106**
high care scores 100–102, **101**, **102**, 107
high health outcomes 103–104, **103**, **104**
vs. long-term expenditures 96
vs. preventative expenditures 96–97

D

'deaths of despair' 5, 31
Deaton, A. 5, 31, 51, 94, 103
'deviant for consistency' 21
'deviant for coverage' 21
directional expectations 37
'disabling profession,' medicine as 93, 95, 96
Dusa, Adrian 19, 38, 76, 157

E

Economist Intelligence Unit 12, 116, 117, 126
education levels 5–6, **6**, 31, 32, 33, **34**, 37, 146
  country clustering **35**, 36
  and health equity **43**, **44**, 45
  and health equity and health outcomes 47, **47**, 48, 52–53
  and health outcomes **38**, **39**, 40, 41, 42, 48, 49, 51
efficiency, health 16–17, **17**
  critique of public sector 67
  directional expectations 71–72
  high 71–72, 75–78, **75**, **77**, 83–85, 86, 142
  high access and high 79–81, **79**, **80**, 85, 86, 87, 142, 146
equifinality 33
Esping-Andersen, G. 3, 149

F

France 91–92, 146
  comparing 10- and 31- country solutions 137, 138
  COVID-19 118
  health outcomes and key causal factors 130, **130**, 131, **131**, 132
  high outcomes (low PYLL measures) 136
  life expectancy *31*
  PYLL and key causal factors **135**
  ranking by health outcomes and PYLL 133, **133**
France, health expenditure **12**, 92, **99**, **100**
  and care score **101**, **102**
  and care score and health outcomes **105**, **106**
  Commonwealth Fund care process score **18**
  Commonwealth Fund health outcomes score **14**
  and health outcomes 103, **103**, 104, **104**, 108
France, health funding **9**, **70**, 91–92

  and access **72**, **73**
  and access and efficiency 79, **79**, **80**, 146
  clustering **71**
  Commonwealth Fund access measure **16**
  Commonwealth Fund efficiency score **17**
  and efficiency **75**, **77**
France, social determinants of health 5, 6, **6**, **34**, **35**, 92
  Commonwealth Fund health equity measure **15**
  Commonwealth Fund health outcomes score **14**
  and health equity **43**, **44**
  and health equity and health outcomes **46**, **47**
  and health outcomes **38**, **39**, 40, 41, 146

G

Germany 54–57
  comparing 10- and 31- country solutions 137
  COVID-19 **119**, **120**, 121, 122, 123, 124, 125, 126, 127
  health outcomes and key causal factors **130**, **131**
  heart disease 49, 56
  high outcomes (low PYLL measures) 136, 137
  life expectancy *31*, 49, 56
  PYLL and key causal factors **135**
  ranked by health outcomes and PYLL 133, **133**
Germany, health expenditure **12**, 56, **99**, **100**
  and care score **101**, **101**, **102**
  and care score and health outcomes **105**, **106**
  Commonwealth Fund care process score **18**
  Commonwealth Fund health outcomes score **14**
  and health outcomes 103, **103**, **104**, 147
Germany, health funding **9**, 55–56, 70, **70**
  and access **72**, **73**, 74
  and access and efficiency 79, **79**, 80, **80**, 87, 146
  clustering 71, **71**
  Commonwealth Fund access measure **16**
  Commonwealth Fund efficiency score **17**

and efficiency **75**, 76, **77**, 78, 84–85, 86, 87
Germany, social determinants of health 5, **6**, **34**, **35**, 57
Commonwealth Fund health equity measure **15**
Commonwealth Fund health outcomes score **14**
and health equity **43**, 44, 45
and health equity and health outcomes **46**, 47–48, **47**, 52, 53, 54
and health outcomes **38**, 39, **39**, 40, 42, 49, 54
Giamo, S. 3
government and compulsory health insurance funding 8, **9**, 63, 67, 68, 141–142
advantages 63
Australia 58–59
Canada 110
disadvantages 63–64
France 91
Germany 54–55, 56
high access 71, 72–75, **72**, **73**, 82, 141–142
high access and high efficiency 79–81, **79**, **80**, 85, 86, 87, 142, 146
high efficiency and 71–72, 75–78, **75**, **77**, 83–85, 86, 142
key causal factor in comparing health systems 129, 130, **130**, 131, **131**, **135**, 136, 137, 138–139
Netherlands 26–27
New Zealand 89–90
Norway 23
Sweden 25
Switzerland 57–58
UK 88, 150
US 9, 69, 112, 148

H

health equity 35, 36, 43–45, **43**, **44**, 51–52, 53, 54, 141
Commonwealth Fund measure 14–15, **15**
directional expectations 37
health outcomes and high 45–48, **46**, **47**, 52, 141
health expenditure 5, 10–12, **12**, 93–114
'care and outcomes paradox' 94, 108–109
challenges in balancing different types of 93–94
curative vs. long-term expenditures 96
curative vs. preventative 96–97

data and expectations 97–100, **99**, **100**
debate around levels of 93, 94–95
high care score and high outcome score results 105–106, **105**, **106**, 108–109, 142
high care score results 100–102, **101**, **102**, 106–107, 142
and high health efficiency 75–78, **75**, **77**
and high health efficiency and high access **79**, 80, **80**, 81
high health outcomes 103–104, **103**, **104**, 107–108, 109–110, 142–143
key causal factor in comparing health systems 129, 130, **130**, 131, **131**, **135**, 136, 137, 138
key findings 142–143
low outcome solutions 147
OECD categories 97–98
outcome measures 17–19, **18**
per capita 8, **9**
primary and secondary care 93
and social determinants of health 18–19, 31, 32–33, **34**, **35**, 36, **38**, 39–40, **39**, 41, 48, 53
health funding 7–9, **9**, 62–92
calibrated data 69–70, **70**
clustering 71, **71**
directional expectations 71–72
high access and high efficiency 79–81, **79**, **80**, 85, 86, 87, 142, 146
high efficiency 71–72, 75–78, **75**, **77**, 83–85, 86, 142
high health access 71, 72–75, **72**, **73**, 81–82, 82–83, 85–86, 141–142
issues and tensions 65–72
key findings 141–142
low outcome solutions 146–147
outcome measures 15–17, **16**, **17**
systems of 62–65
'health gaps' 5, 31–32, 35
Australia 50–51, 60
Canada 111
New Zealand 90
US 113–114
health insurance 7–8, **9**, 63, 64, 67, 68
Australia 59, 60
Canada 110
France 91
Germany 54–55
moral hazard and 66
Netherlands 26–27
New Zealand 90
Norway 23
premiums 64
Sweden 25

Switzerland 57–58
UK 52, 88
US 112–113
see also government and compulsory
    health insurance funding; voluntary
    health insurance
health outcomes 13–14, **14**
    comparing health systems and
        high 128, 129–132, **130**, **131**, 143
    directional expectations 37
    health expenditure and high 103–104,
        103, **104**, 107–108, 109–110,
        142–143
    high care score and high 105–106,
        105, **106**, 108–109, 142
    high health equity and 45–48, **46**, **47**,
        52, 141
    improving through learning 148–151
    key causal factors and high 129–132,
        130, **131**, 143
    low outcome solutions 145–148
    low PYLL and high 134–137
    ranking of countries by PYLL
        and 133, **133**
    social determinants in relation to
        high 35–36, 37–43, **38**, **39**, 48–51,
        53, 141, 146
heart disease 49, 56

I

'iatrogenesis' 93, 95
Illich, Ivan 93, 95, 107
Immergut, E. 3, 62
inequality levels 5, 6, **6**, 20, 33, **34**
    country clustering 34–36, **35**
    high health equity and 43, **43**, 44,
        44, 45, 51–52, 54
    high health equity and health
        outcomes 46, **46**, **47**, 48, 52–53,
        53–54
    high health outcomes and 35–36,
        38–39, **38**, **39**, 40, 41, 42, 48–49,
        50, 53, 143–144, 150
    key causal factor in comparing health
        systems 129, 130, **130**, 131, **131**,
        132, 134, **135**, 136, 137, 138, 139

J

Johnson, J. 22

K

Kuhlmann, E. 1–2

L

Lawson, Nigel 67, 71
life expectancy 30–31, *31*, 95
    Australia *31*, 51, 60

Germany *31*, 49, 56
long-term care health expenditure 11,
    12, 99, **99**, 100, **100**, 101, **101**
    vs. curative expenditures 96
    high care score and high outcomes
        score **105**, 106, **106**
    high care scores 101, **101**, 102, **102**
    high health outcomes and 103–104,
        103, **104**, 107–108, 109–110
    key causal factor in comparing health
        systems 129, 130, **130**, 131, **131**,
        134, **135**, 136, 137, 138, 139
    OECD category 98
    'self-management' of 96
long-term care, systems of financing
    Australia 60
    Canada 111
    France 92
    Germany 56
    Netherlands 27–28
    New Zealand 90
    Norway 23, 24
    Sweden 25, 26
    Switzerland 56, 57
    UK 88, 89
    US 113

M

Marmot, Michael 5, 31–32
McCartney, M. 95
medical goods expenditure
    category 98
methodology, qualitative comparative
    analysis (QCA) 19–22, 87, 151,
    154–164
    calibration 157–164
    consistency 155
    coverage 155–157
minority groupings 30, 32, 33
    Aboriginal and Torres Strait
        Islanders 50–51, 60, 61
    in Canada 111
    Maori and Pacific peoples 90
    in US 113–114
moral hazard 63–64, 66–67
Moran, M. 3

N

National Health Service (NHS) 52, 67,
    88, 149, 150
Netherlands 26–28
    comparing 10- and 31- country
        solutions 137
    COVID-19 **119**, **120**, 122, 125
    health outcomes and key causal
        factors 130, **130**, 131, **131**, 132
    heart disease 49

high outcomes (low PYLL
measures) 136
life expectancy *31*
PYLL and key causal factors **135**
ranking by health outcomes and
PYLL 133, **133**
Netherlands, health expenditure 11–12,
12, 28, 99, **99**, **100**
and care score 101, **101**, **102**
and care score and health
outcomes 105, **105**, 106, **106**, 108
Commonwealth Fund care process
score **18**
Commonwealth Fund health
outcomes score **14**
and health outcomes 103, **103**,
104, **104**
Netherlands, health funding **9**, 27, 70,
70, 146
and access **72**, **73**, 74
and access and efficiency 79, **79**,
80, **80**
clustering 71, **71**
Commonwealth Fund access
measure **16**
Commonwealth Fund efficiency
score **17**
and efficiency **75**, 76, **77**, 78
Netherlands, social determinants of
health 6, **6**, 28, **34**, **35**
CH health outcomes score **14**
Commonwealth Fund health equity
measure **15**
and health equity **43**, 44, **44**, 45
and health equity and health
outcomes 46, **46**, 47, **47**, 52
and health outcomes **38**, 39, **39**,
40, 41
New Zealand 89–91
COVID-19 **119**, **120**, 122, 123,
127
health expenditure 98
health gap 90
life expectancy *31*
Maori and Pacific people 90
ranking by health outcomes and
PYLL **14**
New Zealand, health funding **9**, 70,
70, 90
and access **72**, **73**, 74
and access and efficiency 79, **79**, 80, **80**
clustering 71, **71**
Commonwealth Fund access
measure **16**
Commonwealth Fund efficiency
score **17**
and efficiency **75**, 76, 77, **77**, 78, 84, 86

New Zealand, social determinants of
health 6, **6**, **34**, **35**, 91
Commonwealth Fund health equity
measure **15**
Commonwealth Fund health
outcomes score **14**
and health equity **43**, **44**
health equity and health
outcomes **46**, **47**
and health outcomes **38**, **39**, 40,
42, 146
Norway 23–24
comparing 10- and 31- country
solutions 137
COVID-19 **119**, **120**, 122, 123,
126–127
health outcomes and key causal
factors 130, **130**, 131, **131**, 132
high outcomes (low PYLL
measures) 136
life expectancy *31*
PYLL and key causal factors **135**
ranking by health outcomes and
PYLL **133**
Norway, health expenditure 11–12, **12**,
24, 99, **99**, **100**
and care score **101**, **102**
and care score and health
outcomes **105**, **106**
Commonwealth Fund care process
score **18**
Commonwealth Fund health
outcomes score **14**
and health outcomes 103, **103**,
104, **104**
Norway, health funding 9, **9**, 23–24,
70, **70**
and access **72**, **73**, 74
and access and efficiency 79, **79**,
80, **80**
clustering 71, **71**
Commonwealth Fund access
measure **16**
Commonwealth Fund efficiency
score **17**
and efficiency **75**, 76, 77, **77**, 78, 84,
85, 86
Norway, social determinants of
health 5, **6**, 26, **34**, **35**
Commonwealth Fund health equity
measure **15**
Commonwealth Fund health
outcomes score **14**
and health equity **43**, 44, **44**, 45
and health equity and health
outcomes 46, **46**, 47, **47**, 52
and health outcomes **38**, 39, **39**, 40, 41

O

O'Mahony, S. 93, 95
Organisation for Economic Co-operation and Development (OECD) 7, 9, 31, 64, 68, 95, 103, 116
  health expenditure categories 97–98
  preventative life years lost (PYLL) measure 128
out-of-pocket health funding 7, 8, **9**, 63, 65, 67–68, **70**, **71**, 142, 144, 146
  Australia 60
  France 91
  Germany 55
  high efficiency and 75, **75**, 76, 77, **77**, 78
  high health access and **72**, **73**, 74
  high health access and high efficiency **79**, 80, **80**, 81, 86
  Netherlands 27
  New Zealand 90
  Norway 23
  Sweden 25
  Switzerland 58
  UK 67, 150–151
  US 113

P

personal responsibility for health 64
Pickett, K. 31–32
preventative care expenditure 11, **12**, 99, **99**, **100**
  curative vs. 96–97
  high care score and high outcomes score **105**, 106, **106**
  high care scores 100, 101–102, **101**, **102**, 107
  high health outcomes 103–104, **103**, **104**, 108
  OECD category 98
preventative life years lost (PYLL) measure, OECD 128, 132–134, **133**, **135**
  high outcomes and low 134–137
private health insurance 64
  see also voluntary health insurance
public choice theory 67

Q

qualitative comparative analysis (QCA) 19–22, 87, 151, 154–164
  calibration 157–164
  consistency 155
  coverage 155–157

R

Ragin, Charles 19, 20, 30, 38, 41, 164

rehabilitation services 97
  see also curative and rehabilitative expenditure
Reibling, N. 4
Robert Koch Institute 56

S

smoking 5, **6**, 31, 33, 34, 44, 50
  see also behavioural characteristics
social determinants of health 4–7, **6**, 29–61
  calibrated dataset 34–35, **34**
  country clustering 34–36, **35**
  directional expectations 37
  high health equity 43–45, **43**, **44**, 51–52, 141
  high health equity and health outcomes 45–48, **46**, **47**, 52, 141
  high health outcomes 35–36, 37–43, **38**, **39**, 48–51, 53, 141, 146
  intersectionality 33
  key findings 141
  life expectancy 30–31, *31*
  low outcome solutions 145–146
  outcomes 13–15, **14**, **15**
Sweden 25–26
  comparing 10- and 31- country solutions 137
  COVID-19 **119**, **120**, 127
  health outcomes and key causal factors 130, **130**, 131, **131**, 132
  high outcomes (low PYLL measures) 136
  life expectancy *31*
  PYLL and key causal factors **135**
  ranking by health outcomes and PYLL **133**
Sweden, health expenditure 11–12, **12**, 26, 99, **99**, **100**
  and care score **101**, **102**
  and care score and health outcomes 105, **105**, **106**
  Commonwealth Fund care process score **18**
  Commonwealth Fund health outcomes score **14**
  and health outcomes 103, **103**, 104, **104**
Sweden, health funding 9, **9**, 25–26, 70, **70**
  and access **72**, **73**, 74
  and access and efficiency 79, **79**, 80, **80**
  clustering 71, **71**
  Commonwealth Fund access measure **16**

Commonwealth Fund efficiency
score **17**
and efficiency **75**, 76, 77, **77**, 78, 84,
85, 86
Sweden, social determinants of
health 5, **6**, 26, **34**, **35**
Commonwealth Fund health equity
measure **15**
Commonwealth Fund health
outcomes score **14**
and health equity **43**, 44, **44**, 45
and health equity and health
outcomes 46, **46**, 47, **47**, 52
and health outcomes **38**, 39, **39**, 40,
41, 42
Switzerland 57–58
comparing 10- and 31- country
solutions 137, 138
COVID-19 **119**, **120**, 122, 125
health outcomes and key causal
factors 130, **130**, 131, **131**, 132
heart disease 49
high outcomes (low PYLL
measures) 136
life expectancy *31*
PYLL and key causal factors **135**
ranking by health outcomes and
PYLL 133, **133**
Switzerland, health expenditure **12**, 58,
99, **99**, **100**
and care score **101**, **102**
and care score and health
outcomes 105, **105**, **106**
Commonwealth Fund care process
score **18**
Commonwealth Fund health
outcomes score **14**
and health outcomes 103, **103**,
104, **104**
Switzerland, health funding 9, **9**, 58,
70, **70**, 146
and access **72**, **73**
and access and efficiency **79**, **80**
clustering **71**
Commonwealth Fund access
measure **16**
Commonwealth Fund efficiency
score **17**
and efficiency **75**, **77**
Switzerland, social determinants of
health 5, **6**, **34**, **35**, 58
Commonwealth Fund health equity
measure **15**
Commonwealth Fund health
outcomes score **14**
and health equity **43**, 44, 45

and health equity and health
outcomes 46, **46**, 47, **47**, 52–53, 54
and health outcomes **38**, 39, **39**,
40, 42

T

tobacco 5, **6**, 31, 33, 34, 44, 50
see also behavioural characteristics
truth tables 21–22
Tuohy, C. 3, 110
typologies of health systems 3–4

U

United Kingdom (UK) 87–89
comparing 10- and 31- country
solutions 139
COVID-19 **119**, **120**, 126, 127
health outcomes and key causal
factors **130**, **131**
high outcomes (low PYLL
measures) 136, 137
learning from high outcome
solutions 149–151
life expectancy *31*
National Health Service (NHS) 52,
67, 88, 149, 150
PYLL and key causal factors **135**
ranking by health outcomes and
PYLL **133**
United Kingdom (UK), health
expenditure 12, **12**, 36, 89, 99,
99, **100**
and care score **101**, 102, **102**, 106
and care score and health outcomes
score **105**, **106**
Commonwealth Fund care process
score **18**
Commonwealth Fund health
outcomes score **14**
and health outcomes 103, **103**,
104, 147
United Kingdom (UK), health
funding 9, 70, **70**, 88
and access **72**, **73**, 74
and access and efficiency 79, **79**,
80, **80**
clustering 71, **71**
Commonwealth Fund access
measure **16**
Commonwealth Fund efficiency
score **17**
and efficiency **75**, 76, 77, **77**, 78,
84, 86
United Kingdom (UK), social
determinants of health **6**, 32, **34**,
35, 36, 89

Commonwealth Fund health equity
  measure **15**
Commonwealth Fund health
  outcomes score **14**
and health equity 43, **43**, **44**, 45,
  51–52
and health equity and health
  outcomes **46**, **47**, 51
and health outcomes **38**, **39**, 146
United States (US) 112–114
Affordable Care Act (ACA) 2010 9,
  66, 69, 112, 114, 134, 140, 148
comparing 10- and 31- country
  solutions 139
COVID-19 **119**, **120**
health gaps 113–114
health outcomes and key causal
  factors **130**, **131**
learning from Australia to improve
  healthcare system 148–149
life expectancy 30, *31*
Medicaid 69, 112, 113
Medicare 112
preventable mortality 95
PYLL and key causal factors 134,
  135, 140
ranking by health outcomes and
  PYLL **133**
United States (US), health
  expenditure **12**, 36, 95, 99, **99**,
  100, 113, 147
and care score 101, **101**, **102**,
  106, 107
and care score and health outcomes
  score 102, **105**, **106**
Commonwealth Fund care process
  score **18**
Commonwealth Fund health
  outcomes score **14**
and health outcomes 103, **103**, **104**
United States (US), health funding
  8–9, **9**, 70, **70**, 113
and access **72**, **73**
and access and efficiency 79, **79**,
  80, 146
categorisation 69
clustering **71**

Commonwealth Fund access
  measure **16**
Commonwealth Fund efficiency
  score **17**
and efficiency **75**, **77**
systems 65–66, 67
United States (US), social determinants
  of health 5, 6, **6**, 32, **34**, **35**,
  36, 114
Commonwealth Fund health equity
  measure **15**
Commonwealth Fund health
  outcomes score **14**
and health equity **43**, **44**
and health equity and health
  outcomes **46**, **47**
and health outcomes **38**, **39**

V

voluntary health insurance 7, 8, **9**, 52,
  64, 67, 68, 141–142
Australia 59, 60
Canada 110, 111
France 91, 92
Germany 55, 56
high access and 72–75, **72**, **73**, 82
high access and high efficiency
  79–81, **79**, **80**, 85, 87
high efficiency and 75–78, **75**, **77**,
  83–85, 86
key causal factor in comparing health
  systems 129, **130**, 131, **131**, **135**,
  136, 137, 138, 139, 140
moral hazard and 66–67
Netherlands 26, 27
New Zealand 90
Norway 23
Sweden 25
Switzerland 58
UK 52, 88
US 112, 113

W

Wilkinson, R. 5, 31–32
World Health Organization 3, 7, 50,
  63, 117